KT-525-098

the essential guide to the internet for health professionals

student edition

Sydney S. Chellen

MA (Kent), BA (Ed.), PGCE (FE), RNT, RCNT, RMN, RN

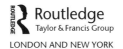

Routledge
Taylor & Francis Group

LONDON AND NEW YORK

First published 2003
by Routledge
11 New Fetter Lane, London EC4P 4EE

Simultaneously published in the USA and Canada
by Routledge
29 West 35th Street, New York, NY 10001

Routledge is an imprint of the Taylor & Francis Group

© 2003 Sydney S. Chellen

The lecturer's photocopiable edition of
The Essential Guide to the Internet for Health Professionals 0-415-22727-X
was published by Routledge in 2000.
It has been completely revised for this non-photocopiable student edition.

Typeset in Optima and Courier by Steven Gardiner Ltd, Cambridge
Printed and bound in Great Britain by St Edmundsbury Press, Bury St Edmunds, Suffolk

All rights reserved. No part of this book may be reprinted or reproduced or utilised
in any form or by any electronic, mechanical, or other means, now known or hereafter
invented, including photocopying and recording, or in any information storage or
retrieval system, without permission in writing from the publishers.

British Library Cataloguing in Publication Data
A catalogue record for this book is available from the British Library

Library of Congress Cataloging in Publication Data
A catalog record has been requested

ISBN 0-415-30557-8

contents

introduction   1

unit 1   health and the net – an overview   5

unit 4 finding health information on the Internet 71

unit 8 publishing on the world wide web 171

unit 9 online help with your health studies and job search 184

twelve big questions and answers 200

appendices 208

worksheets

foreword

Health and social care services are responsible for the delivery of skilled and high-quality care to their patients and clients. Nowhere are these objectives more important than in the fields of nursing, midwifery, radiography, occupational therapy, physiotherapy, health promotion, and social work. And one important quality standard in health care is evidence-based information and best practice. The Internet is a subject on which many people are, let's face it, blissful innocents. I urge you to take the Internet seriously and to discover what is most relevant and useful for your practice – *The Essential Guide to the Internet for Health Professionals* is a practical means towards that end.

The second edition contains new information to help you find your way around the Internet and updates the original book with more detail on the clear framework of the original edition. It's a how-to book to get you going and save you time – a guide to those parts of cyberspace that provide particularly relevant evidence.

Professor Bill Lemmer
Head of Mental Health and Learning Disabilities
Director, Dementia Services Development Centre
(http://dementiacentre.ac.uk)
Canterbury Christ Church University College.

to the reader

to the reader

The **Internet** can be defined as a system that lets thousands of computers all over the world talk to each other.

Windows can be described as a collection of programs, or suite of programs, written for personal computers and published by Microsoft. It is sometimes referred to as a GUI (graphical user interface). There are several versions around: Windows 3.1, Windows95, Windows98, Windows Me, Windows 2000, WindowsNT and Windows XP, the last one being the most recent and most sophisticated.

As a student of health studies or a health professional following a programme in higher education, you will be required to seek relevant information to deliver seminars and write lengthy academic essays. In the past, you would have needed to rely almost exclusively on the resources that are physically on the college campus to acquire this information. The **Internet** has changed all this. It has revolutionized the way students, like you, can enhance their programmes of study. The net has extended the learning resources to colleges, organizations and health experts around the globe, making it unnecessary for you to rely solely on your college library, your college lecturers or even purchasing expensive reference books.

The Internet is a gigantic computer network and you will be surprised how much health information you can uncover (e.g. new drugs, online journals, medical schools, clinical guidelines, consumer health information, and so on). It also offers you the opportunity to share your ideas with other disciplines and empower yourself. Therefore, it is not surprising that there has been an explosion of interest in the Internet since it hit the headlines in a big way in 1994. 'Surfing the net', the 'World Wide Web', 'Information Superhighway' and 'Cyberspace' are all colourful terms that are used to refer to the Internet. Millions of people use it every day, and the number is growing all the time. If you have the appropriate computer system at home, you can even access resources at your college/university (or elsewhere), and obtain limitless information cheaply and quickly.

Despite the mystique surrounding the net, virtually anyone can master the skills necessary to access it. Even if you are new to computers, once you have familiarized yourself with the basic procedures and concepts of using a PC (personal computer) in a **Windows** environment, you too will find it quite easy to use the Internet's many facilities purposefully.

Just take a quick look through the book, and you will see that it has been written for beginners like you. You will also notice that this is not just a book that talks about the Internet and its many wonders: it is a workbook that expects you to practise the skills as you go along. The book has been written in that form because I firmly believe that the only sure way of developing any skill, including Information Technology skills, is to practise. If this is what you feel you require, then this is the book for you.

Information Technology skills are quite complex. Nevertheless, an attempt has been made to split the task into a number of neat 'units' covering different aspects but, to avoid repetition, you will find frequent reference to work covered in earlier units/worksheets in the book. Wherever references have been made to past units or worksheets, look quickly back to the relevant section to remind yourself of what has been covered.

Note As you work through this book you will come across the cue: *Activity. . . .* Worksheets to support certain activities are included. They are an integral part of the work of this book. So follow the instructions given. When you have completed each activity, return to the main text.

Broadly speaking, **software** refers to the programs which provide the driving force of all computing systems. There are two types: Operating Systems software and Applications software.

It should be appreciated that the **software** for using the many facilities on the net may vary from college to college and is in a constant state of change. For the purpose of illustrations and activities, I have chosen a popular network set-up and the most common software likely to be available for use. Even if the set-up and software available in your college/organization or on your home system differ somewhat, you should still be able to benefit from the information in this book and carry out most of the activities set with minimum difficulty. I say this with great confidence as I too have a different set-up at home.

Your overall learning objective is therefore that when you have finished working through this book, you will have met the many inhabitants of the Internet, and will be able to surf the net and use many of its features with a high degree of understanding, competency and satisfaction.

Sydney S. Chellen

about this second edition

In preparing this second edition I have taken the opportunity to rewrite several sections of the book, particularly those in Units 3, 4 and 9, and added new information in Units 5 and 8. Unit 4 has been extensively re-written and contains additional information on search strategies, which include using Boolean logic, planning and steps in undertaking an electronic search. I have also reviewed and updated the list of web sites, worksheets, Appendix 2 (Internet service providers), Appendix 3 (Country codes), Appendix 5 (Glossary of terms) and Appendix 6 (Recommended further reading).

Sydney S. Chellen
Senior Lecturer IT and Research
Canterbury Christ Church University College
e-mail: s.s.chellen@cant.ac.uk

14 December 2002

acknowledgements

I would like to formally acknowledge the support and advice of Karen E. Worden, Subject Librarian at Canterbury Christ Church University College, with the preparation of Unit 4 and related Worksheets. Thanks also to Andy Nazarjuk, Senior Lecturer: Learning Disability Nursing, for providing the set of learning disability web sites and associated review.

I would also like to thank the following reviewers who critiqued the entire manuscript and offered excellent feedback, suggestions and support:

- Mooi Standing, Senior Lecturer: Nursing, Canterbury Christ Church University College
- Eddie Newall, Lecturer: Training and Development, Canterbury Christ Church University College
- Dr Sylvia Prosser, Principal Lecturer: Nursing, Canterbury Christ Church University College
- Keith Jones, Honorary Research Fellow: Centre for Health Services Studies, University of Kent at Canterbury and Network Leader for LASERNET. Formerly Nursing Officer (Examinations Research), English National Board for Nursing, Midwifery and Health Visiting
- Patricia Chellen, School Teacher and Literacy Co-ordinator for Key Stage 2, Napier Primary School
- Students on the BSc Nursing programme
- First-year students on the OT programme
- Radiography students on the MSc programme
- Student nurses on Research modules
- Student nurses on the EN Conversion programme.
- Maurice V. Chellen, LLB, Brunel University.

Dedicated to all the students who put this book to use.

introduction

The Essential Guide to the Internet for Health Professionals is written for health professionals and students following a course in health studies in a college of higher education. Anyone falling into the following categories should find it helpful:

- Students following a Diploma of Higher Education (Nursing Studies);
- Trainee midwives, health visitors, RNs converting to diploma;
- Clinicians following a Bachelor or Master's programme or a path to the Higher Award in nursing, midwifery and health visiting;
- Medical students (doctors, in particular junior doctors and GPs);
- Members of the professions allied to medicine, e.g. trainee occupational therapists, physiotherapists, radiographers, speech therapists, dieticians, pharmacists, paramedics and so on; and
- Those caring professionals who have picked up some cyberspace skills on an ad hoc basis, e.g. nurse lecturers, clinical managers, etc.

how is this book structured?

The Essential Guide to the Internet for Health Professionals is split into nine distinct yet related learning units. It includes the following features:

- **Self-selection of topics/concepts**   Each unit is preceded by a picklist. You are invited to select those items which interest you and are then guided on how to proceed. This picklist provides a means of finding specific answers quickly and easily.
- **Suggested activities and worksheets**   To help you develop specific skills.
- **Appendices**   Containing materials you may find useful later on.
- **Glossary of terms**   A full list of essential terms for quick reference.
- **Recommended reading list**   In Appendix 6, you will find a carefully selected reading list for further knowledge development.

Additional textual information has been included in boxes. Four types of boxes have been used, and they appear throughout the book. Each type of box has been assigned a distinguishing icon to inform you of the type of information being read. They are as follows:

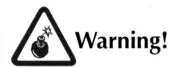

Warning! In this box you will find information to warn you of possible dangers when carrying out certain procedures, or making a decision.

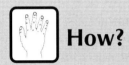

How? In this box you will find information that will guide you to achieve specific objectives.

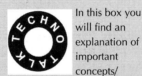 In this box you will find an explanation of important concepts/ technical terms that you might encounter when dealing with a particular area of the Internet.

 Note In this box you will find additional information to clarify a point or information that you might need at a later stage.

conventions used

For clarity, different type styles and keyboard conventions have been used:

CONVENTION	MEANING
Bold	An Internet, e-mail or newsgroup address or part of an address. Text you may need to type into the computer (input text should be typed as it appears).
Bold italic	Text you will type but I don't know exactly what it will be, e.g. a ***keyword***. Text you would click on.
<u>**Bold underline**</u>	A new computer word or expression.
Plain italic	A computer word or expression that has been previously defined and for quick reference can be found in the Glossary at the end of the book.
ENTER (↵)	This means press the ENTER key on your keyboard. N.B. This key might be labelled 'RETURN' or simply have a symbol as shown in brackets here: (↵)

how to use this book

The Essential Guide to the Internet for Health Professionals is self-paced and provides an individualized, interactive learning package. You can read it from cover to cover if you so wish, but you don't have to. You will find that you can dip into any unit or section and learn something. The cross-references adopted in this book should lead/tempt you to other units or sections of the book. When carrying out the activities, it is important that you follow the instructions and apply some common sense. For example, if you find that after having carried out an instruction you do not get the expected result, you should backtrack and try again as you might have done something wrong.

some assumptions

It is assumed that you will have some knowledge of computers and some understanding of Windows, i.e. how to switch on the computer, load Windows and use the mouse. Also that you will be holding the mouse with the right hand. For information in the areas mentioned above, please see a copy of this book: Chellen, S. S. (1995) *Information Technology for the Caring Professions – A User's Handbook.* London: Cassell plc.

what will you achieve?

Each of the units in *The Essential Guide to the Internet for Health Professionals* will help you to develop your understanding of the Internet with opportunities to explore some of its inhabitants, e.g. Gophers, search engines, directories. To give you a feel for the book as a whole, the next page lists the most important learning objectives of each unit.

UNIT	THIS UNIT WILL HELP YOU TO:

1 Health and the net – an overview

Examine the services available on the net and their benefits to students following a course in health studies in a college of higher education.

2 Getting online

Identify the process for getting online on the college computer network. Essential information is included for those of you who want to get on the net at home. This section contains four activities with worksheets to guide you.

3 The world wide web

Identify some important features of a browser and how to use it to explore the web. In this section you will find a selected list of UK and foreign Internet sites applicable to Nursing and allied professions. These sites are organized under thirteen distinct headings as follows:

- Adult nursing and medicine
- Child nursing and medicine
- Learning disabilities
- Mental health nursing and psychiatry
- Midwifery and health visiting
- Medical and paramedical
- Complementary therapies
- Health education
- Health care research
- Journals for health professionals
- Libraries and free health care databases
- Organizations, associations and UK statutory bodies
- Electronic publications and citations.

4 Finding health information on the Internet

Familarize yourself with some of the net's inhabitants. Here you will find eight guided activities (some with worksheets) to help you explore specific Internet databases using effective search strategies to get health information for your projects. In this second edition you will also find discussion and tips on planning a search.

5 Communicating with other health professionals by e-mail

Understand the basics of e-mail and develop skills of using a popular e-mail program. It includes information on e-mail conventions, e-mail overload and other related issues. In this section there are six activities with worksheets.

6 Joining health discussion groups, mailing lists, etc.

Uncover some interesting health newsgroups and mailing lists where you can read messages on a variety of health topics, and participate in online discussions, including real-time conferencing. It will also help you to examine software you need to access news (both at home or at your institution) and discuss relevant issues. Included here are four activities supported with worksheets

7 The gateway to free health and medical resources

Experience using additional tools to make effective use of your net browser. There are three activities supported with worksheets giving you step-by-step instructions.

8 Publishing on the world wide web

Develop an understanding of the design of a web page, and get started in creating a simple web page. There are three activities with worksheets.

9 Online help with your health studies and job search

Locate study tools, evaluate material available on the website electronic sources correctly and use the services on the net to find a job.

unit 1

health and the net – an overview

The development of information processing and retrieval skills, with an ability to operate a computer and produce effective results in letters, documents, and reports, and educational materials, are now very important . . . for ourselves, our colleagues, our students.

E. Ballard (1996)[1]
Senior Lecturer, School of Nursing and Midwifery,
University of Wolverhampton

Many health care students around the world are making it their business to learn how to surf the net because they have realized the wealth of health information it contains, and the opportunity it offers them to share ideas with other students and health care professionals around the world.

The volume of information available via the Internet is huge. Everything that may be of interest to you is scattered around the world on different computers. Collectively these computers make up the Internet. Here is a quick outline of the most popular services on offer that should get you interested:

- **World wide web** – which, among other things, contains a wealth of health information
- Searchable, browsable health and medical **databases**
- **E-mail** for two-way world-wide communication
- **Newsgroups**: a discussion platform of topical health issues
- **Mailing lists** for keeping up to date in your specialist area
- **Internet Relay Chat (IRC)** for distance learning
- **Voice on the net (VON)** for live communication
- **FTP** for looking inside distant computers
- **Archie** for copying files from distant computers
- **Gopher** as an alternative to the web
- **Telnet** to connect your home computer to others on the net
- Easy **publishing** on the web
- **Online help** to assist you, e.g. with your study and jobsearch.

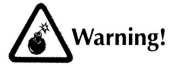 **Warning!** Unplanned surfing of the net, especially at weekends, not only tends to clog servers (computers), but can be quite an expensive activity. A more economical and productive way of using the net is to develop a search strategy. (See Unit 4.)

To view different files on the web, you use web browsing software such as NetScape Navigator or Internet Explorer. Each file (or location) is called a **web page**.

(Also referred to as WWW or the web) is the graphical, multimedia portion of the Internet and is one of the most immediate, easy to use services on the net. It links all the **web pages** together. Thus, a page you're viewing from a computer in Canterbury may lead you to a page in New York, Ottawa, or Sydney with just one click of the mouse. You will find many colleges, universities, libraries, and health institutions, including individual users and others with their own pages (called the homepage). You will be able to read material on almost any topic or any branch of health care. For example, if you have an interest in mental health you can pay a visit to the Mental HealthNet for information on interactive discussion groups, mental health administration tips, popular articles, self-help resources, tools, and information for clinicians. Likewise, if you were interested in Adult or Childcare or Learning Disability you would find appropriate sites. As Howson (1997)[2] puts it:

[Almost] whatever you need to know, you will find a site to answer your question.

(A selected list of UK and foreign web sites applicable to nursing and allied professions is given in Unit 3.) Should you require extra help with your studies, you will find interactive web-based tutorials, which you can explore at your own pace and when it suits you. You will also be able to access some Computer Assisted Learning materials and read up-to-date electronic health journals on a variety of health disciplines. If you learn better by hearing and seeing, then you can watch videos of surgical procedures and look at a vast selection of medical images. (See Units 3 and 4.)

A **database** can be described as a sophisticated electronic filing cabinet capable of storing and sorting large amounts of data in an organized manner. The data can be accessed quickly.

A range of health and medical **databases**, increasingly with full-text services, is being delivered via the Internet. These include bibliographical databases such as Medline or CINAHL and non-bibliographic databases such as the Genome Database. One of the leading electronic information retrieval services is Ovid Technologies Inc. The Ovid-Biomed service provides a fully functional, low-cost Medline service to HE and FE institutions and NHS organizations. The service provides access to important databases, namely: Medline, Cinahl, Cancerlit, Core Biomedical Collection, Ovid Biomedical Collection II, III, IV, Mental Health Collection and Nursing Collection. (The 'Collections' are smaller specialized databases put together by Ovid containing the electronic full text version of up to 20 relevant journals.)

The Ovid-Biomed Nursing Collection offers you the ability to search the database and link from the citation to the full text and print the complete article to take away. It provides access to the following journals from 1995 onwards and is updated on a monthly basis:

- *Advances in Nursing Science*
- *American Journal of Infection Control*
- *AORN Journal*
- *Dermatology Nursing*
- *Heart and Lung*
- *Image: Journal of Nursing Scholarship*
- *Journal of Advanced Nursing*

- *Journal of Clinical Nursing*
- *Journal of Emergency Nursing*
- *Nurse Researcher*
- *Nursing Health Care*
- *Nursing Management (RCN Publishing)*
- *Nursing Standard*
- *RN.*

Note EBMR encompasses two major sources of evidence-based medicine material, the Cochrane Database of Systematic Reviews and Best Evidence.

You will also find that the Ovid-Biomed service has recently included Evidence Based Medicine Reviews (EBMR). This is a useful addition. You can perform a search using medline and retrieve additional information from an EBMR article.

These databases will help you to complete your course assignments. You will be able to interrogate these databases from the comfort of your home or your college computer lab.

It is, however, important to bear in mind that most institutions and organizations – based on the needs of their users and financial constraints – would have selected various combinations of Internet databases to subscribe to. So don't expect to be able to have access to all available electronic databases at your college, university computing laboratory or from your home system. (See Unit 4, Section 4.3.)

1.3 electronic mail (e-mail)

The Internet is a popular communications system that will be around for a long time to come. It brings together the best aspects of postal mail, the telephone, the fax machine, the public/college library, and the newspaper while improving on their worst features. For example, its e-mail service provides you with an easier, cheaper and faster method of keeping in touch. You can use it to collaborate on common projects with health care students in places like the US and Russia, or simply exchange personal messages with other health care colleagues, friends or relatives at other networked sites almost anywhere in the world – without the need to use paper, pen, envelope, stamp and post box. By drafting and sending e-mail to foreign health care students you will be able to increase your range of communication skills and extend your use of language. Although most e-mail messages are just ordinary text, you can attach almost any type of computer file you want to send along with it (such as a spreadsheet, word-processing document or even a picture), and encrypt the message so that no one except the intended recipient will be able to read it. When working in the community you will be able to quickly and efficiently transmit files and data 'back to base' or to other health care professionals from a portable or notebook computer, whilst on the move. By sharing information in this way you will help to enhance the quality, responsiveness, targeting and efficiency of health care in the NHS. (See Unit 5.)

1.4 newsgroups

These are discussion groups and each focus on one particular subject. The discussion itself takes place through a form of e-mail, but the major difference is that messages are passed around the whole group to read, and added to. There are hundreds of health groups you can join, such as nursing, midwifery, medical informatics, pharmacy, radiology, and many more. If you like sharing your views with other health care students or health professionals, you will find the Usenet newsgroup irresistible. It provides a forum for discussion of issues related to a wide range of specialist subjects. Here you will be able to engage around the clock in group discussions, exchange information and ideas with other health professionals all over the world and seek information from them. This is a great and fun way to test your thoughts on particular health issues. (See Unit 6, Section 6.1.)

1.5 mailing lists

Mailing lists are available in many areas of health and medicine. They offer yet another way for students, researchers, lecturers, and clinicians to discuss key topics with fellow professionals. The mailing list is a special kind of e-mail address that re-mails all incoming mail to a list of subscribers on the mailing list. Mailing lists differ from newsgroups in that a separate copy of the mailing list message is e-mailed to each recipient on the list. Each mailing list has a specific topic, so all you need to do is to subscribe to the ones that interest you. (See Unit 6, Section 6.2.)

1.6 internet relay chat (irc)

This is a novel, but unfortunately expensive way to communicate in 'real-time-typing'. Nevertheless, here you can hold conversations with one or more health professionals by typing messages back and forth that instantly appear on the screens of everyone involved .(See Unit 6, Section 6.3.)

1.7 voice on the net (von)

If your computer has a soundcard and a microphone plugged into it, you can talk to anyone in the world just as you do with a telephone (provided they are online and have a soundcard and microphone too). Since your Internet call will be a local call, you may be able to hold conversations at a cheaper rate than using a telephone. In the not too distant future you will be able to access tutors over a two-way real-time video link between the college and clinical areas. (See Unit 6, Section 6.4.)

1.8 file transfer protocol (ftp)

Note

FTP is one of many protocols used to copy files from one computer to another on the Internet. Also used are terms like 'an FTP site' (a site that lets you grab files from it using this protocol).

The collections of computers that make up the Internet hold a combined library of millions of files. The **FTP** system lets you look inside directories on some of these computers and copy files straight to your hard disk just as if you were copying files between directories on your own computer system. (See Unit 7, Section 7.1.)

1.9 archie

Copying files from a distant computer to your own using FTP is quite simple, but first you have to track down the file you want. If the file exists, Archie will help you find it in seconds. All you will need to do is to enter the name of the file (or part of it) into a program that can search through indexes of files on computers on FTP sites. (See Unit 7, Section 7.2.)

1.10 gopher

If you are happy with the World Wide Web you may not be at all keen on Gopher. Nevertheless, Gopher is an older Internet filing system. It is menu-driven and offers an alternative way of searching, retrieving and reading materials from local and remote sites on the Internet. Although, since the arrival of the World Wide Web, Gopher's popularity has been on the decline – leaving a reduced number of links to Gopher sites – you should still find many useful documents stored on Gopher servers. (See Unit 7, Section 7.3.)

1.11 telnet

Telnet provides a facility that will let you connect from your home computer to another computer, for example your college computer, across the Internet and use it as if you were directly connected to it. This can be quite useful if, for instance, you need to search your college/university library catalogues for available books. (See Unit 7, Section 7.4.)

1.12 publishing on the net

Anyone can become an author on the Internet. You will be able to use the web to publish articles or results of a research project you have completed. You may even be interested in launching your own newsletter or web page. (See Unit 8.)

1.13 online Help with your health studies and job search

Online is a synonym for 'connected'. Anything connected to your computer and ready for action can be said to be online. In Internet terms it means that you have successfully dialled into your service provider's computer and are now connected to the net. The opposite term is offline.

Online classes are slowly appearing. At some web sites you will find information about examinations, tips for success, summaries for syllabuses and so on. You will also find useful web sites to help find a job in the health care profession. (See Unit 9.)

There are many more things to do on the net that makes it so compelling to 'surf'. In fact the Internet is the place to learn more about the Internet.

In this book I will tell you step-by-step how to get online using your home or college computer, how to find your way around and how to use most of the services mentioned above. I will show you how to use literature searching and evaluation strategies to access the information you need for your course assignments from Internet databases. I will also show you how to use the net to locate and correspond via e-mail with experts in your field, and to join chat groups plus more.

There is a wealth of health information on the net. As a whole it has many users, but the world wide web is the most popular and e-mail is growing in use all the time. There are many different ways of getting the information, some more expensive than others, but once you have the knowledge to use them, you can choose the best way for you.

unit 2

getting online

getting online

The hardest thing for me was getting started, but once I was hooked-up I just could not get off. I have splashed out on a computer system, and I go online every evening, checking my e-mail box and participating in newsgroups.

Student on Project 2000
Canterbury Christ Church University College, Kent

 Account is a term used in computer science to describe a record-keeping arrangement employed by a System Manager at a college, university or health organization, and a vendor of an online service. It helps vendors to identify their subscribers, for example, for billing. System Managers of multi-user systems use it to identify their users for administration and security purposes. A personal computing account is rather like your bank account. This has a password (i.e. a secret code used to keep things private) that 'only' you know, together with an account name (Username) that identifies you.

Username is a unique name you are assigned by a service that enables you to connect to it and identify yourself, demonstrating that you are entitled to access it.

Getting online is another way of saying getting connected to the Internet. You can get online in several ways. However, as a health care student or clinician registered for any part-time or full-time course at a university or college where computing facilities with Internet connection are in place, all you will need to start surfing the net is an **account**. Then, as long as you remain a student at that college and you comply with your user agreement (see **Appendix 1**), you will enjoy unlimited free access.

However, if you would like to surf the net in the comfort of your home you will need the appropriate bits and pieces. This Unit will help you to identify the process of getting online at the college. You will also find essential information on the equipment you need to get on the net at home. A brief explanation of computer hardware and accessories are given along with suggestions you may find useful when deciding to purchase a computer.

checklist

Below is a checklist of what you can expect to find out in this Unit. Read through the statements then tick (✓) the items about which you would like to know more.

I would like to find out more about:

Please now read through the topics you have ticked.

You cannot get a *Username* and *Password* until an account has been set up for you. This done, you can use your allocated Username and Password to access the computer, get on the net and do many of the things outlined in Unit 1.

How?

how to obtain a college computing account

Once you are a fully registered student on a course of study, you will normally be given information about the computing facilities available, where they are, how to obtain a personal computing account, what to do should you need technical help, and so on. If this has not happened in your case, you should contact your personal tutor and/or Computing Services department and someone will set up an account for you. In some colleges you will find a system of self-registration is available. If you use virtually any PC in the computing laboratories or an Open Access Area for this purpose. The self-registration procedure is usually quite simple. After registration you usually will need to wait 24 hours before you can log on the network.

2.1.1 nine ways to help you protect your password

As a health care student, at the end of your course you will probably join a hospital Trust, where, as part of your daily work, you will be using a computer system containing data about patients. It is, therefore, vital that from the start you get into the good habit of taking extra care of your *Username* and *Password*. Start practising good habits during your period in college/university. There are several strategies you can use to keep your password safe. Here are nine of them:

9 ways to help you protect your password

1 Never type your password in front of another person where (s)he can see the keys you press.
2 Never use swear words because they are easier to guess.
3 Never use the following as a password: your username, the name of the computer you are logged into, the name of your department, or words such as 'PASSWORDS' or 'SECRET', because they are words that immediately come to everyone's mind.
4 Never use any word, name or number that has an obvious association with you personally, such as your own name or nickname, name of your spouse, partner, boyfriend, girlfriend, name of your child or pet, your own date of birth or that of a member of your family, your car registration number, your telephone number, or name of the town in which you live.
5 Never choose a plain English word or a personal name as a password – because a '**hacker**' can write a program that runs through a computerized dictionary trying every word as a password.
6 Always change your password on a regular basis – normally the computer system will force you to change it periodically.
7 Always change your password if you suspect that it may have been discovered by someone else.
8 Always keep your username and password secret – avoid writing it down.
9 Always choose a password that will lodge in your mind so that you will not need to write it down. For example, use unusual words at least six characters long combining letters and numbers such, as 12blue.

Hacker is a term normally used to describe a skilled programmer who invades systems and ferrets out information on individual computer access codes through a process of trial and error.

2.1.2 choosing and remembering a password

When choosing a password you should always make sure that it will be easy for you to remember and difficult for others to guess. Here are a few suggestions for you to consider:

- Select the first letter of each word of your favourite proverb, catchphrase or song, e.g. **IHSSIWF** (I Have Started So I Will Finish); **YSFT** (Your Starter For Ten)
- Select two colours and join them together, e.g. **redblue**
- Select a significant year and spell some of the digits, e.g. **10SIXTY6** or **TEN66**
- Select an English word you use a lot and add a two-digit number before or after it, e.g. **18LOVE** or **LOVE18** (the number could be the first or last two numbers of your telephone or year of birth)
- Select two words which are the opposite of each other, e.g. **YESNO**
- If you have been allocated a password that you can't change, you can make it easier to remember by creating a mnemonic. For example, if your password is **wkj11** you could remember it as **Willie King John the eleventh**.

2.2 getting started with the college computing system

Windows NT is a true multitasking, multithreaded 32-bit operating system for IBM or IBM compatible PCs that are connected to a network. It has increased power and stability, but it not quite as *user friendly* as Windows 95 is.

Once an account has been set up and you are in possession of a working username and password, you are ready to log on to the Internet. All you now need to do is go to a computer lab and sit down comfortably in front of a **Windows NT** workstation. Before doing the next activity, here are a few words about the rules that you must obey, at all times, when using college computing facilities.

2.2.1 regulations governing college computing facilities

All colleges, universities and Trust hospitals that provide computing facilities will have 'regulations' governing their use. The full text of these regulations will have been issued to you or may simply be displayed in computing laboratories and perhaps in certain other places. It is usually deemed to be your responsibility to read these regulations and to ensure that you comply with them. Failure to adhere to the rules could lead to your being banned from using the network and disciplinary action taken against you. By way of example, I have included in **Appendix 1** a typical User agreement that you can expect from colleges and universities, when you register to use computing facilities.

Activity 2.1   logging on and off your college computer system

Using a Windows NT workstation, log on to the system. You will need to enter your allocated *Username* and *Password* when requested.

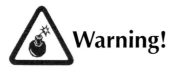

Warning! If you have difficulty logging on, you should seek help from the Helpdesk at your institutions, otherwise you will not be able to use your college system to get on the net, nor will you be able to carry out the other activities in this book.

Once you have logged on successfully, familiarize yourself with the Windows environment including making sure you know how to log off properly.

When you have completed the activity return to this page and read on.

2.3 getting started with a computing system at home

There will be times when you would wish you could work on your health projects or other course assignments and do your literature search while sitting in the comfort of your home. You now can and it need not cost you an arm and a leg. As mentioned already, to get *online* at home you first need a few bits and pieces. You may already have a few of them. Carry out Activity 2.2 below – this inventory will help you determine your current position.

Activity 2.2   equipment needed to surf the net at home

A **modem** is a device that converts data back and forth between the formats recognized by computers and the format needed to send it down the telephone line.

Service provider is a general term for a company that gives you access to the Internet by letting you dial into its computer. This may be an Internet service provider (ISP) or an online service provider (IOP). For additional information see Section 2.3.5.

Here is a list of what you will need to start surfing the net at home. Use this checklist to tick (✓) your requirements.

Checklist:
- ☐ A computer
- ☐ A **modem** to use with your computer
- ☐ A telephone line to connect your modem
- ☐ Communication software to drive your modem
- ☐ Membership of a **service provider** to get on the Internet
- ☐ An electronic name and address (this will be issued to you by the service provider, when you join a service)
- ☐ The electronic name and address of the person you are attempting to communicate with.

Below you will find some information about each of the bits on the checklist above that you might find useful.

IBM (short for International Business Machines) is an American computer manufacturer, with headquarters in Armonk, New York. The company is a major supplier of information-processing products in the United States and around the world. Its products are used in a wide variety of industries, including business, government, science, defence, education, medicine, and space exploration.

A **laptop** is a type of computer light enough for you to use while resting it on your lap and because it weighs around 9 to 12 pounds it can also be carried around.

A **desktop** computer as the name suggests is kept on top of a desk or any suitable hard work surface.

To **download** is to copy files (of any type) to your own computer from some other computer. The opposite term is to upload.

RAM – an acronym for Random Access Memory. It is a temporary storage space for information you are currently working on. Information stored in RAM is lost when the computer is switched off.

There are several families of computers on the market. Almost anyone with a computer will be up to the task. However, the health care Trusts and most colleges and universities use **IBM** or IBM-compatible computers. It will therefore make good sense to opt for one of those. There is also the question of whether you should opt for a **laptop** or **desktop**. Here are a few suggestions that you might find useful when making a decision to purchase a computer.

- **Laptop** vs. **desktop** – Unless you plan to travel a lot with your computer, you will be better off with a desktop. This is purely and simply because you will pay less for the same performance.
- **Speed** – Faster models are coming out almost every year. The Pentium range of computers is quite fast. These are fitted with different types of Pentium chips. Some Pentium chips are faster than others. The speed at which a chip can process information is measured in megahertz (MHz). The slowest Pentium chip works at 60Mhz and the fastest (at the time of writing) is 2G550Mhz. Processor speeds could well reach 3GHz by early 2003. (Waiting to be released is the next generation of processors, the Intel Itanium and the AMD Sledgehammer.) Although you do not need the fastest chip in your computer to surf the net, I can assure you that the faster the computer, the more likely you are to enjoy your online search and the longer it is likely to serve you. So go for the newest and fastest model you can afford.
- **Windows** – Windows 95 has built-in support for Internet connections that make all the setting-up easy. Windows 98, ME or 2000 makes connections even easier as they include Microsoft's own browser: Internet Explorer. The latest arrival, Windows XP, tops the lot.
- **RAM** – When surfing the net, there are times when your computer will need to be able to temporarily remember lots of information at once. The amount of random access memory (**RAM**) available in your computer will matter. The more RAM memory there is, the more information your computer will be able to remember simultaneously. RAM, which is measured in megabytes (MB, where 1024 kilobytes [KB] equals 1 MB), is limited by the amount that your machine can support and you can afford. As programs are getting bigger, 64MB of RAM is becoming the absolute minimum in a new machine. However, you should consider at least 128MB or even 256MB.
- **Hard disk** – This provides a place to store software programs along with any information that you may have in RAM and want to keep. The hard disk is a vital piece of hardware, as you will need to install a few new programs to get on the net. You will also require storage space if you plan to download some of the free software available on the net. Hard disks come in two main varieties: IDE (Intelligent Drive Electronics) and SCSI (Small Computer System Interface). Hard disks tend to fill more quickly than you would think, especially after you've been online for a while and have accumulated an impressive health care library of your own. Most new desktop machines come with a minimum of 10 gigabytes (GB) of hard disk space, more than enough for Internet use. If you plan to **download** a lot of images, get one with 30 GB hard drive or larger. A gigabyte is about 1,000 megabytes.
- **Sound card** – If you would like to use Voice (see section 6.4) and hear musical offerings on the net, then you'll need a sound card. There are various types. An example is a 32-bit AWE sound card by Creative Labs.

Refresh rate is the rate the electrons scan the screen. Your computer measures this rate in hertz (Hz). The higher the hertz, the better. In addition to the rate, you may see a note saying the monitor is interlaced (scans only every other line) or non-interlaced. However, interlaced monitors can flicker, so you will probably want to get a non-interlaced monitor.

Dot matrix is a fairly basic but flexible printer. It can produce text or graphics in the form of a matrix of small dots, with each character formed by a series of pins striking a ribbon. They are generally used for jobs where the quality of the printing is not crucial.

Inkjet printers can be described as the 'poor man's' laser printers (see below). The inkjet printing system prints characters and graphics by firing ink drops at the paper from thin nozzles. These printers use replaceable ink cartridges that contain both the print heads and the ink.

Laser printers are fast, flexible and sophisticated devices that produce high-quality printing. They work on similar principles to a photocopier, using a photosensitive drum, and can produce between 4 and 20 pages per minute.

CD-ROM stands for 'Compact Disc Read-only Memory', which is a disc used for storing and distributing large volumes of data.

- **Monitor** (VDU or Video Display Unit) – This is a critical component of your computer system. As you will be staring at the monitor for long hours when surfing the net, you must get a good quality monitor. There are important standards to look for. The most important are: Resolution, Size, **Refresh rate**, Memory, Bus type, Knobs and Swivels. Activity 2.3 will help you identify the quality of the monitor you have or are planning to have.
- **Keyboard and mouse/track balls** – Keyboards have a fairly standard layout, but they do differ in terms of ergonomics and feel. There are many types of mouse, and each one feels different. The keyboard and the mouse are the two items you will use to give instructions to the computer. When surfing the net you will probably use the mouse most. So get yourself a good one, that you feel comfortable with. If you have difficulty using a mouse, you may want to consider a Track ball instead. This is like an upside-down mouse with the roller ball exposed. To make a movement, you roll the ball itself.
- **Printer** – Strictly speaking you do not need a printer to surf the net. But if while trawling the net you find useful information to complete your health project or other assignments, to print out your find you will need a printer. As can be expected a variety of printers exist, but really there are principally three types to choose from. Here they are in order of increasing quality and cost: **dot matrix**, **inkjet** and **laser**. For most work you should find inkjet quite adequate. Here is a checklist of other factors to consider:
  - Speed
  - Colour or black and white output
  - Running cost
  - Noise level
  - Paper handling
  - Size.
- **CD-ROMs** – Many databases (in the private or public domain) are now available on **CD-ROMs**. CD-ROM is a recent innovation for literature searching. It combines the great storage capacity of optical compact discs with computer database software to give you a fast and efficient method of compiling a list of references. Almost all libraries these days have a selection of commercial databases on CDs. Thus if your PC is fitted with a CD-ROM drive, you may be able to borrow these CDs to use in the comfort of your home. The slowest drive available at the time of writing was the 6-speed (sometimes noted as 6×), and the fastest at present is 52-speed. Don't buy anything slower than a 12-speed. 24-speed upwards should be acceptable. The faster the quoted speed of the CD drive, the faster it will read data from the CD, making your life easier.

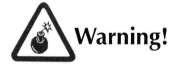

Warning!

Regardless what you might hear, CDs are not indestructible. While they might survive a fall, a misplaced fingerprint on the silver data-surface might make some of the data unreadable. So always handle CDs by their edges, and keep them in their case when you're not using them.

If the CD needs cleaning, wipe it gently with a soft cloth. Always wipe in straight strokes from the centre to the edge of the CD.

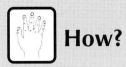

How?

how to retrieve a stuck cd

If a CD gets stuck in the drive and the tray won't eject, find a paper clip and straighten it out, insert it into the tiny hole in the front of the drive unit and push. The tray will slowly slide out. If the tray won't close by pushing the button after you've removed the offending CD, push it gently back into the unit and restart your PC as soon as you can to let the drive reset itself.

Activity 2.3 which vdu?

Note TFT screen (i.e. flat screen) is becoming popular but the price remains high and is not likely to drop until 2005, but (according to computer magazines like *PC Answers*) some dealers may well offer you a 15-inch TFT screen as an alternative to a 17-inch monitor. A choice well worth considering.

To enjoy the World Wide Web you will be happiest with a display unit that has the following spec or better. Use this checklist and tick (✓) the specification (spec) of the monitor you have or are planning to buy.

Checklist:

☐ A VGA monitor which can display 256 colours with a resolution of 800×600 or an SVGA 256-colour monitor with a resolution of 1024×768

☐ 17-inch screen

☐ A screen refresh rate of 70Hz

☐ 2MB video card

☐ VESA (Video Electronics Standards Association) or PCI (Peripheral Component Interconnect) bus

☐ Non-interlaced scanning

☐ Has touch-buttons or knobs to adjust settings such as brightness, contrast, etc. and . . .

☐ Has a stand that swivels so that you can adjust it.

2.3.2 which modem?

Note . . . if you already have a computer that does not measure up to the specs I have suggested, you may still be able to use it to get on the Internet. However, if it is more than two years old, think twice before upgrading it. You might be better off selling it and buying a new one.

Your *modem* is one of the key links between your computer and your Internet service provider. The other link is your telephone line. Two of the most important features to look for when choosing a modem are speed and compatibility. The faster the modem, the quicker it will move information from one end to the other, thus reducing the cost in your telephone bill and online charges. The best you can get in a two-way modem using ordinary phone lines is 33,600 bits per second (bps). (A new technology called ×2, lets you download information at 56,000 bps from specially equipped Internet service providers.)

Modems typically connect between your computer and your telephone line. However, if you have cable Internet service available in your area, then you will find a cable modem a worthy alternative. These units plug into your cable television outlet and allow you to download data at up to 1.5 million bps – 25 times faster than the fastest telephone modems. However, there is a hefty monthly service charge attached to it.

Although you can get by with a 28,800 bps modem, you will find it slower. So, if you are buying a new phone modem and can afford it, go for a 33,600 bps modem with ×2 capability. However, do make sure you check the connection speed offered by your service provider. If you decide to go for cable modem, get the one your cable TV company recommends.

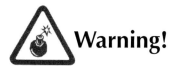

Warning!

incoming calls and call waiting

. . . if someone picks up an extension phone while you are logged in, it usually breaks your connection.

. . . if you have call waiting you should turn it off while your modem is on the phone. For touch-tone phone type *70, (don't forget the comma) in front of the number of your Internet service provider in your communication software. If you have a pulse-dial phone type 1170, before the phone number.

Note BT is offering anyone with a PC and ISDN card a new service called **Home Highway**. The advantage of this service is that it enables you to use both the phone and the Internet with a single BT connection. For additional information on Home Highway please turn to Question 8 in the section Questions & Answers.

2.3.3 which type of telephone line?

You can use your ordinary single telephone line to connect to the Internet, but it must have a plug-in socket. The socket must be located fairly close to your computer. Using an adaptor, you should be able to plug-in the modem and a telephone in the same socket. If you want people to still be able to phone you when you are surfing the net, then you will be wise to have a second telephone line.

ISDN line – If you really need faster access to the Internet, you can get an ISDN line. This stands for Integrated Services Digital Network. It is a different type of link to your Internet service provider. It replaces your modem with a new device called a 'Terminal Adaptor' and it can operate at four times the speed of a 33,600 bps modem. Right now it is very expensive and complicated. Cable modems may make it obsolete.

2.3.4 which communication software?

Communication *software* (or *comms program*) enables your computer to communicate and exchange information with other computers that are linked by *modems*. There are several types of comms software. For example, *Windows95* comes with Exchange and HyperTerminal while *Windows 3.1* comes with Terminal. When you purchase your modem it usually comes with its own comms software. Also, major service providers like Freeserve supply their own comms software.

If you bought your computer from a dealer stating that the system is 'Internet ready', then everything would have been done by the person who installed the software. However, if you have or are planning to install a modem on your own computer, then you will need to set up the software yourself or get someone else to do it for you.

2.3.5 which internet service provider?

Finally, you need to find a way to connect to a computer that is part of the Internet. The service provider is your gateway to the net.

So what is a service provider? Several hundred large companies in the UK maintain networks that are linked to the Internet via dedicated communication lines. Many of them are willing to let people like you and I use their dedicated communication lines to access the Internet, typically free of charge. The

Note Shell account vs SLIP or PPP account. Direct connection such as SLIP or PPP lets you download files directly to your system from remote sites. While with indirect connection such as a Shell account, when you download a file from an Internet site the file is saved on the service provider's computer. You then have to transfer the file from the service provider's computer to your home system.

SLIP (short for Serial Line Internet Protocol) and **PPP** (short for Point-to-Point Protocol), are Internet standards for transmitting Internet Protocol (IP) packets over serial lines (phone lines). Internet information is packaged into IP packets (a method for enclosing data into small, transmissible units wrapped up on one end, unbundled on the other). A service provider might offer SLIP, PPP, or both. Your computer must use connection software (usually provided by the service provider) that matches the protocol of the server's connection software. PPP is a more recent and robust protocol than SLIP. So if you have a choice, select PPP.

company you choose to log to the Internet is your service provider. Selecting which service provider is right for you may not be that easy, but is nevertheless a decision that you will have to make. These days Internet service providers can be divided into three types: online (subscription) services, '0800' ISPs and 'Free' and (local) Internet service providers.

- **Online services** – This type of service provider offers much more than basic Internet access and consequently charges more. Online services are like an exclusive club. Once you sign up you will have access to a range of members-only areas such as discussion forums, chat groups and file libraries as well as access to the Internet. You will also have user-friendly interface, special features unique to that provider, better security, longevity, and lots of user support. See **Appendix 2** for a brief outline of the major players. Online services sound pretty good, but it could cost more than you are willing to pay. Read on, as there are other alternatives.
- **'0800' Internet Service Providers (ISPs)** – Here you pay a fixed fee for the service and you get unlimited access in return. See **Appendix 2**.
- **('Free') Local ISPs** (also called 'pay-as-you-go') – The two most popular kinds of accounts are Terminal or UNIX shell accounts and SLIP/PPP accounts.
  - *With a terminal or UNIX shell account*, your computer does not interact with Internet computers. You dial into your service provider's computer to indirectly connect to the Internet. Shell accounts are limited in features but less expensive than direct access accounts.
  - *With SLIP or PPP account*, you dial into a service provider's computer and run applications that directly connect you to the Internet. With this kind of direct connection your computer can use browsers with user-friendly graphical interfaces, such as NetScape, Internet Explorer or Eudora to interact with Internet computers. **SLIP** or **PPP** access to the Internet offers more performance and convenience than a shell account and cost a bit more.

Here are a few reasons to consider ISPs:

- Lower cost; many providers offer a flat monthly rate (plus your telephone bill, of course)
- Choice of tools to access the Internet, e.g. Microsoft Internet Explorer, NetScape, Eudora, and so on
- Less censorship
- You can normally choose the personalized part of your e-mail.

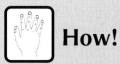

How!

how does an account with a service provider work?

The ISP provides you with a dial-up phone number. This phone number is called PoP (Point of Presence) (Fig. 2.1). Using the software provided you dial-up the number to establish a link and the ISP routes you into the Internet.

Large Internet service providers have several PoPs. These are scattered across the country, thus providing users the facility of access using local calls, while others have only one PoP which may not be close to you.

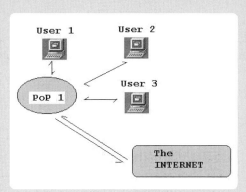

Fig. 2.1 An illustration of a PoP

2.3.6 taking out a subscription

Note Remember, there is no such thing as a perfect service provider – all of them are good for some people, bad for others. It is perfectly reasonable, therefore, to try several services before picking the one you like best.

Recently, service providers like the Sun, PC World and a few others have started to offer free access to the Internet. They are able to offer this because instead of charging you and me a monthly subscription they get their fund from three sources, namely:

- A percentage of the cost of your phone call whenever you connect to the net
- Revenue from advertisers and
- The 50p to £1 they charge when you call their help lines for assistance.

There are loads of ISPs (Internet Service Providers) and a few online services in the UK. New ones are popping up all the time. Check the business pages in your local newspaper. For your convenience I have listed some of these providers in Appendix 2.

Choosing a provider can be a skill in itself. There are a few things to consider and a few questions to ask. Good service providers will be willing to provide you with straight answers. Here are ten key-points to guide you.

10 points to consider when choosing an ISP

1 **Charges** – You need to ask yourself a few questions, such as are you prepared to pay for a good service that gets you online every time and gives you lots of information and content? If so, you should try a subscription service. But do check for hidden charges. For example, do they charge extra for the time you spend online, as you'll need to take this into consideration. Do you go online occasionally and want to pay as little as possible? Then try a 'free' ISP (sometimes called 'pay-as-you-go' – usually at local rate via your phone bill). Do you want unlimited access for a fixed fee so you can budget for it? Then find out which 0800 service fits you.

2 **Connection** – Seek past or present subscribers' opinions as to the reliability and availability of the system, especially during peak periods.

3 **Location of the PoP** – Enquire if the computer you are dialling into (the PoP) is local. Since the largest single cost you will face in using the Internet is your telephone bill, it's very important that you choose a provider who has a PoP as close to you as possible. If you are not able to dial-in using a local phone number, then forget it and try another provider.

4 **Modem speeds** – Check the speed of the modem the service provider is using. If you have a fast modem, e.g. 33.6Kbps, you do not want to connect to a service provider who uses a slower modem.

5 **PPP connection** – Enquire if you can choose PPP connection as opposed to SLIP connection. The former is faster and easier to set up.

6 **E-mail address** – If you want more than one e-mail address for different members of the family, then check this first. Most ISPs should offer several.

7 **Personal website** – Do you want to have your own website? Check that the ISP gives free 'webspace', and how much. 10 MB should be enough for most sites, but if you're ambitious you might want a service provider who gives more.

8 **Software** – Many companies will send you preconfigured connection software that's ready to install. Ask about availability of technical telephone support if you get stuck.

9 **Subscription fees** – Find out the monthly subscription fee (if any), inclusive of VAT. If this ISP charges more, ask what else they provide that other companies don't. Enquire if you can pay annually, as this may be cheaper.

10 **Support** – Ensure that there is appropriate support for your system. (If you are an IBM user, you should expect your provider to offer wholehearted support for IBM Internet applications.) Also, check that good telephone support is available and whether there is a charge, particularly when you are most likely to need it, i.e. during evenings and weekends.

2.3.7 signing up

On taking up a subscription with a provider, you will be given an account name. Providers differ in their approach to account names. Some just assign you a name, while others allow you some degree of choice, as long as the name has not already been used. It is important that you choose an account name that you like, because your account name will often form the unique part of your e-mail address, and this is the way you will be known to the rest of the world. Also you will need to quote your account name when you call the support line. So try not to ask for names, like 'chubbychops'. While this may seem funny at first thought, you may regret it later on when you're using e-mail to apply for a job.

There are two or three common approaches to choosing an address. It's worth following these, as they're accepted as 'normal' on the Internet.

- The first approach is your initial(s) followed by your surname. For example, mine is '**sschellen**'
- The second approach is your initials, e.g. '**ssc**'. Had there already been an 'ssc' on the system, a number can be added, e.g. '**ssc1**'
- The third approach is your main forename followed by the first letter(s) of your surname, e.g. '**sydc**'. If this already exists on the system, then it could be '**sydch**'.

Most providers are reluctant to change people's e-mail addresses after the account has already been set up. So a few minutes of thought beforehand can avoid a lot of hassle later.

The rules on account names vary a little between providers. Usually they are lower-case, can't contain spaces, and are often restricted to eight characters. Most importantly, another subscriber must not have already chosen it.

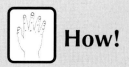

How!

how do you get an account for a system at home?

For your home system, once you have chosen your Internet service provider, get on the phone and tell them you would like to subscribe. The provider will then set up an account for you. What happens next would vary from provider to provider.

- They may send you an account, followed by a disk preconfigured for your computer with instructions for installation.
- They may send you a disk of software, written instructions on how to install it and how to configure your computer, and some useful documentation.

If you have decided to subscribe with an online service provider, your first job is to get your hands on a free connection software. Phone them and request the correct software for your computer (see Appendix 2 for telephone numbers).

If a disk is supplied, somewhere on it you will be told how to start the program that signs you up, and the whole process will advance in simple steps.

Usually you will be able to try the service for 30 days. After you have keyed in all required details, the program will dial-up the service's computer and automatically set up your subscription. After a few minutes you should receive a username and password.

how do I use an online service?

When you dial-in to your online service and log on using your username and password, you won't actually be on the Internet. You will find the main screen displaying a series of buttons. To access the Internet, you will need to click on a button clearly labelled Internet.

2.4 JANET and the web

U-NET limited is one of several Internet service providers. It is a service that is aimed solely at Windows users.

e-mail: hi@u-net.com

WWW: http://www.u-net.com

Tel: 01925 633144
Fax: 01925 850420
For a list of other ISPs refer to
Appendix 2.

As mentioned already JANET (Joint Academic Network) is the academic network of UK universities. It is designed for academic use by staff and students. As a health care student you are eligible to apply for a JNDS (JANET National Dial-up Service) account with **U-NET**. It is a service seriously worth considering. So, before you rush out to take a subscription with any ISPs or online services, you should enquire at the Computing Services department of your college about a JNDS account. If you already have a JNDS account, you should be able to do at least five things. Activity 2.4 will help you to identify them.

Activity 2.4 checklist for a jnds account

Here are the five things you should be able to do with a JNDS account, for an annual flat rate fee with no hourly charges or time limits. Use the checklist to tick (✓) those that you can do.

☐ Pick up your college/university e-mail from home;
☐ Access and surf the net for all kinds of information;
☐ 'Chat' directly to other Internet users;
☐ Obtain high-quality, high-speed access to JANET to do your research or other projects from the comfort of your home;
☐ Use 5Mb of webspace – for your hobbies, CV or other pleasures.

If you are able to do all the above and possibly more, you are doing well. Otherwise, you should have a serious chat with the service provider. You should also be provided with all the software you need to get online, calls at local rate, technical support in the evenings and on Saturdays, and you should have a choice of e-mail addresses that you can take anywhere and keep after you leave education.

summary and conclusion

You will need an account to get online. Once you have obtained this, you must guard your password. If you are using your college/university NT workstation, this gives you free unlimited access to the net, so use it as much as you can. If you are purchasing your own PC then go for the higher-end machine within your buying range, especially the modem. After you have chosen a good Internet service provider you are ready to surf away.

unit 3

the world wide web

Before I knew how to use the Internet, I was always behind with my projects because I just could not find the books I needed in the library. But, I can tell you this: the Net is so unbelievable. Now that I have access to so much information, I am never late with any of my assignments.

Student on Diploma of Education (Nursing Studies)
Canterbury Christ Church University College

The World Wide Web is one of the most immediate and easy-to-use services on the Internet.

Howler (1997)[3]

Patients will increasingly approach health professionals with information they have gathered from the web. It is vital therefore, that practitioners know which sites are reliable and valid sources of information and how to guide patients to them.

Cooper (2001)[4]

URL (pronounced 'earl') is the unique 'address' of a file on the Internet.

A **browser** is a computer program that enables you to view web pages on the Internet. Although the NetScape browser was very popular, Microsoft Internet Explorer has become more popular, particularly with home users.

The main advantage of Internet Explorer is that Microsoft gives it away for free. Although you can now get a copy of NetScape Navigator free of charge it is unlikely to retain the popularity it previously enjoyed. It is worth noting that there are things that NetScape Navigator can do and Internet Explorer can't, and vice versa, but in general they are equally powerful.

The world wide web ('web' or 'www', for short) is so easy to use that it has become the most popular service on the Internet. It is probably the reason for the 'Internet explosion'. To access the information on the web you need a piece of software. NetScape Navigator is one of two major software programs that do the job well. The other major competitor is Internet Explorer. In this book, the screenshots have been taken from Internet Explorer* as this is the browser which home users are most likely to have on their system. One of the big advantages of the web is that you do not need a menu. You use the hypermedia links embedded in web documents to thread your way through all types of related information. You can also access any document you want directly by entering its location through a **URL** (Uniform Resource Locator).

In this unit we will identify some important features of a **browser** and how to use it to explore the web.

*The Internet Explorer program used for this book was provided by Freeserve, hence the FS logo on the top right-hand side of all screenshots.

Below is a checklist of what you can expect to find out in this Unit. Read through the statements then tick (✓) the items about which you would like to know more.

I would like to find out more about:

Please now read through the topics you have ticked.

Hypertext is a system of clickable texts used on the web. These clickable texts serve as a cross-reference to another part of the document (or an entirely different document).

The web, developed by CERN (European Laboratory of Particle Physics) in Switzerland, is a system that uses the net to link together vast quantities of information all over the world. It is made up of a series of 'pages', containing both text and graphics. Some of the words or phrases are underlined and highlighted in a different colour from the text around them. These are called **hypertext** or hyperlinks. If you place your mouse-pointer on to one of these hyperlinks (you'll see it change into a hand with a pointing finger) and click the mouse button, you will be transported to either a new section of the text or a brand-new document.

Note A web page is a single document that can be any length, like a document in a word processor. Pages can contain text, graphics, sound and video-clips, together with clever effects and controls.

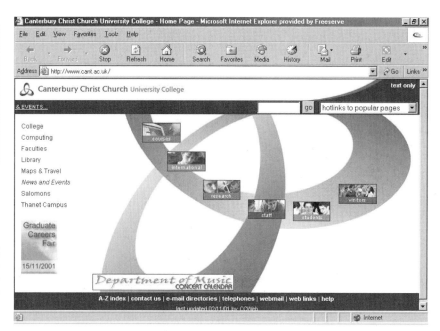

Fig. 3.1 A web page showing hyperlinks
By moving your mouse-pointer over coloured hypertext and clicking your mouse-button, you can jump between pages of related documents

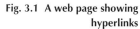

Note The 'web' is developing all the time, and is likely to become the biggest library on earth – an invaluable resource for any health student doing research or completing course assignments.

Here are a few points to remember about these two features of web pages:

- Hyperlinks are not restricted to opening documents stored on the same computer. You could be reading a page stored on a computer in Kent and clicking a hypertext could take you to a page stored on another computer in Australia.
- Hypertext links are not always a word or phrase. Sometimes there is a picture that you click on, or a part of a larger picture, with different parts linking to different pages.
- Besides opening a new web page, a link sometimes would display a picture, download a program, play a video or a sound, run a program and so on . . .

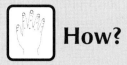
How?

recognizing a link
Text links are quite easy to recognize because they are underlined and in a different colour. A picture link may not be quite so noticeable. However, you can move your mouse-pointer onto the picture. If it is a hyperlink, you'll see your pointer change into a hand with a pointing finger.

3.1.2 storage of web pages

Web site is a term loosely used to refer to web pages belonging to an individual or organization. A site could be a single page or several complex pages belonging to a university, college, hospital Trust or a Nurse Therapist.

The web is made up of many millions of files placed on computers called web servers. Although no one person or company owns the web itself, the web servers are owned by different companies. They either rent or give away free space to anyone who wants to put their own pages on the web. These pages are created using a text-based language called HTML (HyperText Markup Language). Once these newly created pages are available on the web, anyone who knows their address can read them.

Simple web pages can be created in minutes. Thus, a **web site** can be as up-to-date as its creator wants it to be. Some are updated more frequently than others.

3.1.3 web browsers

Note . . . students from other institutions can visit CCCUC by entering this website address in the Address/Location box: http://www.cant.ac.uk

As already mentioned, to view pages on the WWW and information from other Internet resources, you'll need to use a browser. The browser that you use determines how the web information is displayed. Some browsers provide a text-only feature and cannot display the richer content of web files that may include graphics, video or audio clips. There are a number of these available. No matter which browser you use, you will be able to access thousands of research sources to complete your health projects. The only things you might miss are the effects of multimedia presentation. In this book we will concentrate on Microsoft Internet Explorer for two reasons: first it is a browser, that is now quite popular, especially with home users, and second, it is the one that is likely to become the standard in most colleges.

When the browser is activated the first page is loaded and displayed on the screen. This starter-screen is known as the 'homepage'. A homepage – like the one shown in Fig. 3.2 – serves two purposes: it allows the college to present an image of what the institution is about, and it lets you and other students and staff establish links to other sites of interest. For example, in the Canterbury Christ Church University College (CCCUC) homepage you will find hyperlinks to various pages created by the college, and to other web sites around the world. If you are not at CCCUC, the homepage at your institution will look different and will provide a completely different set of links since each site's homepage defines the links it feels are most appropriate.

3.1.4 starting your browser

Address or **Location** box is the box where you type your favourite web site addresses. In Internet Explorer this box is labelled 'address' while in NetScape Navigator it is labelled 'location'.

Before you can start using some of the features on your browser you must first be connected to the Net. This is fairly easy to do in a Windows environment if you are able to use a mouse. It is just a matter of identifying the appropriate icon and double-clicking on it with your mouse. If you are not sure how to gain access to the net, the next activity will help you do so. When you reach the homepage, take a good look at your browser and make a special mental note of the **Address** or **Location** box.

logging on and off the internet on a college network

I am assuming in this book that you have the program, 'Microsoft Internet Explorer' or 'NetScape Navigator/Communicator' installed on your WINDOWS NT WORKSTATION. If this is the case, follow the step-by-step instructions listed in Worksheet 1, they will help you get on and off the Internet. Please complete both the logging on and off.

If you're using NetScape Navigator/Communicator or something else, you should find that most of the facilities available on Microsoft Internet Explorer are also available in other browsers, and many of them can be accessed by similar toolbar buttons, menu options or keystrokes.

When you have completed the activity return to this page and read on.

 Warning!
If you are unable to identify the Microsoft Internet Explorer icon to start the program (or the icon of the browser installed on the system you are using), you should seek help immediately. You should find the Help desk in your institution quite accommodating.

Worksheet 1 logging on and off the internet on a college network

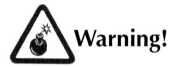

NetScape icon

Internet Explorer icon

Starting your browser

1 Log on to Windows NT now (if you have not already done so).
2 Identify the **NetScape** or **Internet Explorer** icon.
3 Using the mouse, **double-click** on the icon. *This should start the browser program and – if all goes well – the homepage of your service provider (or your institution) should be loaded and displayed on the screen.*

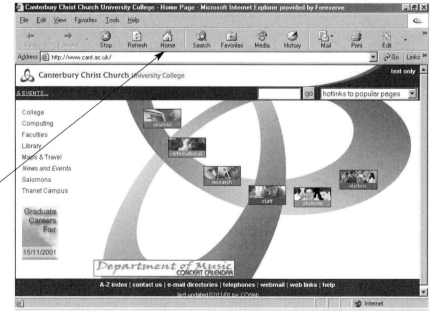

Fig. 3.2 The homepage of Canterbury Christ Church University College

Comment
Don't worry if what you see on your screen looks slightly different to the screenshot on the left. The homepage is where you will start exploring the web. You can return to the homepage at anytime by clicking on the '**Home**' button on the tool bar.

Quitting the Internet

1 Point and click on the command **File**. *A submenu should appear.*
2 Point and click on the command **Close/Exit**. *You should be back to Windows Program Manager or Windows Desktop.*

Comment

You have just arrived online, and you are eager to explore. There are a few things more I need to tell you before you start your adventure. So let's get off the net for now and continue reading Unit 3. To quit follow the steps on the right.

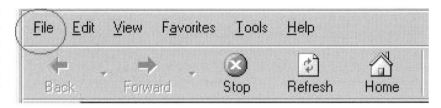

3.1.4.1 some important features of internet explorer and netscape browsers

Although there are a number of browsers (some available in several versions), most share some common features.

Note

Having carried out Activity 3.1 above, you would have noticed the homepage displayed by your browser. It may have resembled in some way the homepage in the screenshot below. You may also have noticed some of the features of your browser and of the web page. These may not have made much impression on you. However, they are features that you will be using over and over when exploring the web and surfing the net. So let's get acquainted with the basic workings of a browser and the web itself.

Fig. 3.3 Some important features of a browser

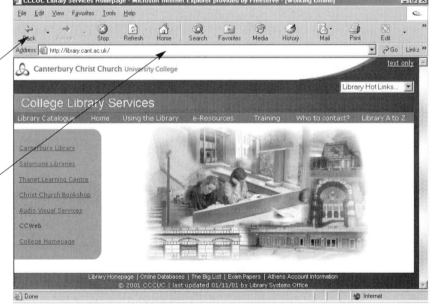

Comment

Buttons on the toolbar allow you to navigate between pages, point you to interesting places and enable you to refresh a web page's content. Most of the buttons on the Internet Explorer also appear on NetScape Navigator.

Comment

This white box shows the address of the current page. It is also the box where you can type your favourite web addresses (URLs). In *Internet Explorer* this box is labelled 'Address' while in *NetScape Navigator* it is labelled 'Location'.

If you look at the homepage shown above you should be able to see several *hypertext links* (i.e. underlined, coloured text). When you move your screen-pointer onto any link and click on it, your browser sends a message to the server storing the page that you have requested. Then, if everything goes according to plan, the server responds by sending back the requested page so that your browser can display it. Links that you have visited before are (usually) in red; those which you have not visited are (usually) in blue. Figure 3.4 shows another screenshot. We can use this as an example to highlight the type of thing you will find on a web page, which are as follows:

- **Plain text** – This is ordinary readable text. Clicking on it will have no effect.
- **Plain image** – A picture or graphic that simply enhances a web site and it won't lead anywhere if you click on it.
- **Hypertext links** – Text links to other places ('hotlinks'). Text links are nearly always underlined and their text colour is usually red, after they have been visited. Clicking on these will route you to a related topic.
- **Hyperlink images** – These do the same thing as hypertext link. In most cases they look no different to ordinary images, but they may be outlined in red or blue or the same colour as any hypertext links on the page.
- **E-mail link** – Click on this link and you will be able to send an e-mail message to the web page's author. The author's address will be automatically inserted into the message for you.

Fig. 3.4 Some elements that make up a web page

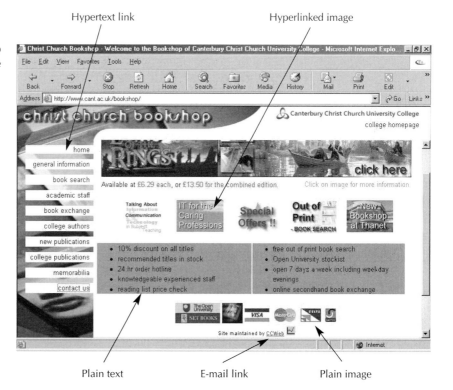

Hypertext link   Hyperlinked image

Plain text   E-mail link   Plain image

Every page on the web has its own individual address (URL: Uniform Resource Locator), which tells your web browser where to find it. The standard format used for specifying the desired URL is composed of four simple components that identify the critical elements needed to access a document. Below is the URL of a government department: it is the homepage of the English Department of Health. Incidentally, it has details of, among other things, the Health of the Nation plus updates and research findings.

Let's use the URL http://www.open.gov.uk/doh/dhome.htm to examine the four components.

Table 3.1
The components of a URL

Transfer format	Host computer	Directory path	Filename
http://	www.open.gov.uk/	Doh/	dhome.htm
1	2	3	4

Hosts are computers that are directly connected to the Internet.

1 In Table 3.1, the first part of the URL is the transfer format. It indicates a hyper-text (i.e. a web page) and tells your browser the transfer format that will be needed. (Table 3.2 shows some common transfer formats.)

2 The second part of the URL is the name of the **host** computer on which the web page is stored. Note that it is separated from the transfer format by a colon(:) and two forward slashes (//).

3 The third part of the URL is the directory path on the host computer where the web page is stored. Note that the components of the directory location are separated from each other with a single forward slash (/), not the back-slash (\) that some other operating systems expect.

4 The fourth and final part of the URL is the name of the file containing a hypertext document. In our example it is the homepage of the Department of Health in the United Kingdom. Web documents are usually given the extension **.html** or **.htm**.

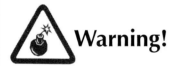

Warning!

It is important that when typing a URL you match capitalization and spelling in any component correctly. The slightest typing error will prevent your browser from fetching the document you requested.

When an Internet link like the one above does not work, try entering just the root of the address, i.e. 'the transfer format' and the 'host computer'.

Most URLs start with 'http://', which means that they are ordinary WWW addresses (the 'http' stands for 'Hypertext Transfer Protocol', which is the system NetScape uses to fetch WWW pages). There is an older and simpler service that you may find, called 'Gopher'. (For additional information read Section 7.3.) You may encounter Gopher sites if you look at university information systems; Internet Explorer and NetScape are quite happy to handle them. The URL of a Gopher site will begin with 'gopher://'. It's also possible to use your web browser to access anonymous FTP sites (see Section 7.1), in which case the URL will begin with 'ftp://'. There are a couple of other service types – especially Usenet news ('news:'), or e-mail ('mailto:') (for additional information read Unit 6).

Transfer format specification	Server accessed
http://	World wide web
https://	WWW with secure links
gopher://	Gopher
ftp://	FTP
news:	USENET
mailto:	e-mail

Table 3.2 Common transfer formats

The following is a short list of other mysterious things you will see in URLs:

- **.html** or **.htm** is the filename extension for a hypertext document
- **Index.html** is the master page of a web site
- **.Txt** is a plain text document without links
- **.Gif** or **.jpg** or **.jpeg** is a picture
- **www** is short for world wide web.

3.1.8 domain names

Note Host and domain names are important because they can help you to infer something more about new resources as they are discovered. For example information from a UK organization ought to have more authority than one located on a US organization computer.

Every site on the Internet, whether accessed by WWW, e-mail, FTP, etc. is addressed by the Internet 'domain name'.

A domain name is composed like an address on an envelope. It consists of several parts strung together with full stops ('dots'). Domain names are usually decoded from left to right. In the URL we looked at above, the domain name is:

http://www.open.gov.uk

The **.uk** shows that the site is in the UK. A site in Denmark ends with **.dk**; a site in China ends with **.cn**. An Australian site uses **.au** or sometimes, for historical reasons **.oz**; a site in India ends with **.in**. Some domain names don't end with a country code: these are usually (but not always) in the USA. There is a **.us** domain, but it's not often used – the Americans don't put their country on their domains for a similar reason to why we in the UK don't put the country on our stamps – they were there first. Also United Kingdom uses uk instead of the country code GB. Appendix 3 offers a comprehensive list of countries that have Internet connection and their country code.

The next domain, in our example above, to the left is **.gov**, which indicates a government institution (sometimes they use **.govt**). A commercial organization uses **.co**, a similar US site would use **.com**. An academic organization such as a university would use **.ac** (or in the US, **.edu**). A school uses **.sch**, a non-profit organization uses **.org**, and backbone Internet organizations use **.net**.

Anything to the left of the organization name is up to the organization to assign – in the example above, the **www.open** identifies the particular computer within the organization, which handles the World Wide Web.

3.2 navigating the web

When you view a web page using your browser, you will see that it contains information and 'hotlinks'. These are usually underlined, as shown in the screenshot below. To follow the hotlink (i.e. a key phrase or word) you simply place your mouse-pointer on it and click the mouse-button.

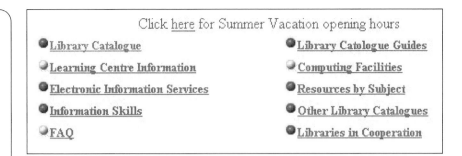

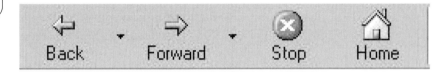

A link you've visited before will be displayed in a different colour (usually red rather than blue). Also, most web pages will have more information in them than can be seen comfortably on a screen. Use the 'scroll bars' at the right and underneath the page to move up and down and left and right within a page.

With these buttons located on your browser's toolbar you can retrace your steps.

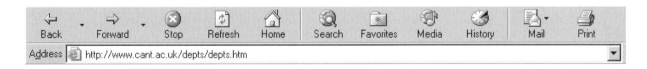

For example, you can click on the '**Back**' button to go back a page or more. When you have gone back, you can click on the '**Forward**' button to go to the next page again. To return to the Homepage, simply click on the '**Home**' button.

Your browser keeps track of the pages you have visited in your current session. At any time you can go back to an earlier page by clicking on the '**Back**' button located on the toolbar and return to a later page by clicking on the '**Forward**' button.

While pages are being fetched you will be entertained by a lightning storm around the 'Internet Explorer' or 'NetScape' icon. Fetching pages can take quite a long time – especially from overseas. At busy periods the Internet can get swamped, and at these times you may lose patience with the slow speed at which, for example, pictures can be retrieved. Just point and click on the '**Stop**' button to interrupt your browser.

3.2.1 internet explorer toolbar

In Activity 3.2 below you will be navigating the web. You will no doubt notice a few more features on your browser's toolbar and wonder about their functions. The browser you are most likely to use is Internet Explorer or NetScape. So, here is a quick comparison and review of both of them.

Fig. 3.5 The Internet Explorer toolbar and address box for typing URLs

Table 3.3 lists the 12 buttons shown above along with a description of each and also compare the buttons with that found on NetScape toolbar.

Back	Forward	Stop	Refresh	Home	Search	Favorites	Media	History	Mail	Print

Address http://www.cant.ac.uk/depts/depts.htm

Table 3.3	Button	Internet Explorer	NetScape
Description and comparison of toolbar buttons on two popular browsers	**Back**	Clicking this button will take you back to the last page you looked at If you keep clicking you can step all the way back to the first page. If you don't want to go through them all, the downward arrow to the right of this button will bring up a menu listing those pages. Click on the one you want.	Takes you to the page visited. Hold down the mouse button and you'll get a list of previously visited sites.
	Forward	After going back, you can go forward again (to the next page you looked at) with this forward button. This button will be greyed-out if you haven't used the **Back** button yet. The downward pointing arrow to the right of this will bring up a menu of all those pages you visited.	Takes you forward to a more recently visited page. Hold down the mouse button to get a list of those sites.
	Stop	At busy periods it could take a long time before a page is loaded. If you have lost patience, click on the '**Stop**' button to interrupt Internet Explorer.	The same as '**Stop**' on Internet explorer. It stops a web site being loaded.
	Refresh	Sometimes things go wrong. Click this button and Internet Explorer will start downloading the same page again.	On NetScape Navigator this button is labelled '**Reload**'. It does the same as '**Refresh**'.
	Home	As explained already, the homepage is where you will start exploring the web. You can return to the homepage at any time by clicking on the '**Home**' icon. If you used a CD-ROM to install your Internet Service Provider it's more than likely that this will have set the ISP's own website as the homepage. You can change your homepage by going to '**Tools**', on the bar above, then clicking on 'Internet **Options**' and typing in the address of the website you want your browser to open on.	Takes you to your homepage.

Table 3.3 (cont.)	Button	Internet Explorer	NetScape
	Search	Clicking '**Search**' on Internet Explorer 5/6 will open a search engine in a separate window on the left-hand side of the screen. Here you can type in what you want to find, hit **Enter**, and the search engine will look for websites about that subject. Clicking on the link to that website will bring it up in the main screen.	This button opens up NetScape's own search website – Excite.
	Favorites	Like '**Search**' clicking '**Favorites**' will open a separate window on the right-hand side of the screen, with a list of your favourite sites organized into folders. You will need to store these yourself, but sometimes your installation CD will put some in for you.	In NetScape this button is called '**Bookmarks**'. Similar to Favorites on Internet Explorer. Clicking on '**Bookmarks**' it brings down a list of your favourite sites.
	Media	Click this '**media**' button brings you the Media bar. This bar makes it easy for you to play music, video, or multimedia files. You can use the Media bar to listen to your favourite Internet radio station while you use your computer.	
	History	Click on this icon and you will see a list of all the sites you have visited. Generally those you have visited previously. In most cases clicking on it you should be able to revisit these sites offline.	
	Mail	This opens a menu from which you can run your e-mail or newsreader software, or open a blank form to send an e-mail message. A quicker way to get to Outlook Express.	
	Print	Prints the current page. A dialogue box lets you select printing characteristics.	
	Edit	If you're interested in designing your own webpage and come across a website you particularly like, clicking on '**Edit**' will let you look at the programming behind that site.	

	Button	Internet Explorer	NetScape
Table 3.3 (*cont.*)	**Address bar**	Where you enter the address of the website you want to visit. Just click in the space, type in the address, such as the one here, and click on '**Go**' or press **Enter** on your keyboard.	On Netscape this Address bar is called '**Location**'. Type the address of the website you want to visit and press **Enter** on your keyboard.
	My-Netscape		This is Netscape's main advantage over Internet Explorer. Clicking on '**MyNetscape**' opens up your own personalized webpage. Click on '**Personalize**' on this page to enter your details and preferences, and Netscape will set up a page customized to your needs, including the news you're interested in, a personal calendar, horoscope, and a direct link to your e-mail.
	Security		Another useful button, especially when shopping online. Click '**Security**' to find out if the page you are viewing is 'secure' (i.e. if other people can view it).

Activity 3.2 exploring the web

Internet
Explorer
icon

NetScape
icon

Now that you know a few things about your browser, let's start using it to make an initial exploration of the web.

- The step-by-step instructions listed in **Worksheet 2** should help you to follow a few links and to skip from page to page casually. If you find yourself going down a blind alley, use the tools *'Home'*, *'Back'*, *'Forward'* and *'Stop'* discussed above to retrace your steps, and move in a different direction.
- If you are an absolute beginner to the Internet, don't try to overdo it on this initial visit. Contain yourself to using the tools discussed so far.

When you have completed the activity return to this page and read on.

Worksheet 2 exploring the world wide web

Charting your course
1 Log on to Windows NT as you did before.
2 Identify the **Internet Explorer** or **NetScape** icon.
3 Using the mouse, **double-click** on the icon. *This should start the browser program and – if all goes well – the homepage of your service provider (or your institution) should be loaded and displayed on the screen.*
4 Point and click on any hotlink you want to explore.
5 Now, follow the hotlink and other hotlinks until you are ready to stop. Practise using those buttons on your toolbar: **Back**, **Forward**, **Stop** and **Home**.
6 When you are ready to finish, close down your browser and log off Windows.

3.2.2 address or location box

'URL' is just a convoluted term for 'address'. You might have already noticed that the URL of the current page is shown in the 'Address' or 'Location' box. Every time you open a new page, its URL appears in the Address/Location box.

If you know the location (i.e. the URL) of a page, you can go directly to it. You simply type it into the location box and press the Enter key (on your keyboard). For example, if you are interested in oncology and need information on cancer you can go directly to the Cancer Oncolink site by typing this URL:

http://cancer.med.upenn.edu

At this site you will find information on many different types of cancer and the latest treatment, and much more.

In the next Activity I will give you a few URLs to enter and you will be able to follow up some useful sites.

3.2.3 hotlists

As you work with the Internet sites, you are going to discover places that you will want to revisit frequently. Rather than typing the address each time you need to access the site, you can add it to a list and your browser will remember this list between sessions. Internet Explorer refers to this hotlist as **Favorites** while NetScape Navigator calls it **Bookmarks**. The steps for creating a hotlist are quite easy. The next activity will show you how to do this. But first, here is the process (Fig. 3.6).

Fig. 3.6 How to create a hotlist

Creating a hotlist in Internet Explorer

1 Select '**Favorites**' on the menubar. *A dropdown list should appear.*

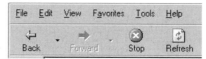

2 Select the command '**Add to Favorites**' from the list to add the current page to your Favorites list.
3 Click on the **OK** command.

Internet Explorer allows you to organize your shortcuts into submenus to make them easy to find. You simply select the file or files, then click one of the buttons to organize them.

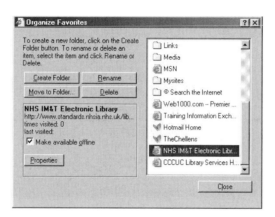

Creating a hotlist in NetScape Navigator

Select '**Add Bookmark**' from the Bookmark menu to add the current page to your bookmark list

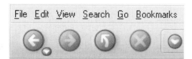

Netscape's Bookmarks window allows you to drag elements in your bookmark list around, and insert headers and separators.

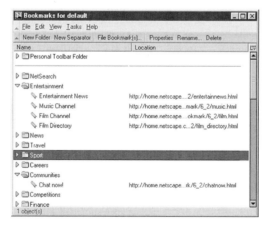

If you select an element in the Bookmarks window and choose '**Properties**' from the '**Item**' menu, you get this window which allows you to rename the bookmark and add notes.

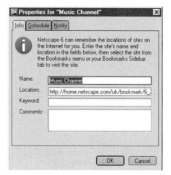

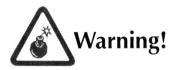

Warning! When you try to open a web page you may experience problems. For example, at the time you requested a page, the server may not be running or it may be busy. In both cases your browser may respond with a message 'Time out', and in the latter case you may get a part of the page and then everything seems to have stopped. In the case of the latter, you may be able to get things moving by clicking the **Reload** (**Refresh**) button on your browser's toolbar. This will get your browser to try again. This may be sufficient to solve the problem, but be prepared to give up and try again later. There is also the problem of the 'vanishing page syndrome'. Although all web pages contain links, sometimes the pages those links refer to no longer exist and you will receive an error message instead. This is because the web is constantly changing, hence pages (or even sites) move elsewhere, are renamed, or simply disappear. So, some of the URLs included in this book may have expired by the time you get to try them. This is, unfortunately, part of the magic of the web.

3.2.4 exchanging hotlists

Both Internet Explorer (I.E.) and NetScape Navigator keep your hotlist in a folder/file on the hard disk. The folder in I.E. is called '**Favorites**' and is stored in Windows directory; while in NetScape Navigator the file is called '**bookmark.htm**'. Both files can be read by other web browsers.

If you want to send your hotlist to a friend, this is not as difficult as you may think. Simply locate and copy the file onto a floppy disk or if you want it to go by e-mail, enclose it as an attachment (see Unit 5 on e-mail).

Both browsers have the ability to import any **.htm** file, extract the hotlinks, and put them in your Favorite/Bookmark list. Thus if while surfing the web you find a list of links which interest you, just save the page as a .htm file by using the '**Save As . . .**' option from your browser.

Now that we have covered a bit more about the WWW, you should have sufficient understanding of it, and how to navigate your way around with a reasonable degree of confidence and satisfaction. So let's try another activity.

Activity 3.3 entering URLs and adding interesting sites to your hotlist

- Read **Section 3.3**, taking special notice of the caution given in the warning box.
- Select a few sites you would like to visit.
- Use the step-by-step instructions in **Worksheet 3** and start trying out all or at least some of the web addresses you have selected from the list offered.
- Add those sites you want to revisit later on to a hotlist (for help refer to **Worksheet 4**).

When you have completed the activity turn to the next page and read on.

More and more sites of interest are emerging all the time. Once you become familiar with the net you will no doubt discover all the sites you care to discover. You will find bloated volumes of directories of web sites in your library or bookshop. You will also find some web pages listing interesting web sites. I have gathered a list of useful UK and foreign sites and organized them under the following thirteen headings that you should find helpful when searching for information for your coursework.

- Adult nursing and medicine
- Child nursing and medicine
- Learning disabilities
- Mental health nursing and psychiatry
- Midwifery and health visiting
- Medical and Paramedical (include radiology and occupational therapy)
- Complementary therapies
- Health education
- Health care research
- Journals for health professionals
- Libraries and free health databases
- Organizations, associations and UK statutory bodies
- Electronic publications and citations.

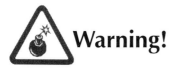 **Warning!**

Each of the sites listed in this book have been checked on several occasions to ensure there have been no changes to site addresses since this book was written. As the web is still growing, it is possible that some sites might restructure their information as they add new areas of content. If you find an address to which you could not connect, you should try connecting to the host system without specifying a particular document for viewing. In other words, if the site in the book is listed like this:

http://www.scilib.uci.edu/~martindale/HSGuide.htmL

you might try connecting to this address:

http://www.scilib.uci.edu

You can then look through the main content areas at the site to see if you can find the information in a new location.

Worksheet 3 uniform resource locators (URLs)

The Internet is growing all the time. Russell (1998)[5] reports that over 100 new WWW sites are added each day. In Section 3.3, I have listed a series of URLs of Internet sites for nursing and the allied professions which you can visit and evaluate their usefulness for yourself. All you will need to do is to type any chosen URL into your web browser's Address/Location box and press the Enter key on your keyboard. See steps below.

Entering URLs

1 Log on to Windows NT and then start your Browser. After a few seconds the homepage should appear.

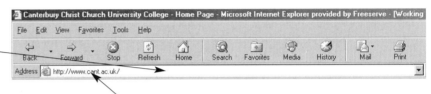

Comment

One way of clearing the content of the Address/Location box is as follows.

Place your mouse-pointer in the box and double-click on the (left) mouse button. This should highlight the content of the box.

Then press the **Backspace** key on your keyboard. The content of the box should vanish.

2 Clear the content of the Address/Location box.

3 (Select a URL from Section 3.3) or if you have one of your own, type it as shown in the screenshot on p. 43.

4 Make sure there are no typing errors, then press the Enter key (on your keyboard). If all goes well, after a while the requested page should load.

5 If you are absolutely sure you have typed the address correctly and have still received an error message, click on the '**Home**' button on the toolbar and try another address.

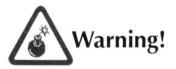

Warning!

Remember that fetching pages can take a long time especially from overseas, and also at busy periods. So, be patient. If you are tired of waiting, point and click on the '**Stop**' button on the toolbar. Then try another address.

Worksheet 4 adding a web site to a hotlist

For Internet Explorer

ADDING FAVORITE

1 Point and click on the command **Favorites** on the menubar. *A submenu should appear.*

2 Click on **Add to Favorites**. *An Add Favorite dialog box should appear.*

3 Click on the **OK** button. *The Add Favorite dialog box should disappear, and the URL of your current web page would have been added to your Favorites.*

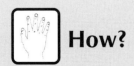

How?

To check that the URL of your current web page has indeed been added to your Favorites list, first click on the '**Home**' button. Then click on the command '**Favorites**' on the toolbar, and you should find a reference to the page you have stored. To load that page again, simply point and click on it.

For NetScape Navigator

ADDING BOOKMARK

1 Point and click on the command **Bookmarks** on the menubar. *A submenu should appear.*

2 Click on the command **Add Bookmark**. *The submenu should close, and the URL of your current web page would have been added to your bookmark list.*

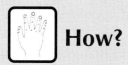

How?

To check that the URL of your current web page has indeed been added to your bookmark list, first click on the '**Home**' button. Then click on the command '**Bookmarks**' on the toolbar, and you should find a reference to the page you have stored. To load that page again, simply point and click on it.

adult nursing and medicine

Deaf and Hard of Hearing
http://www.hearingconcern.com/

This site provides information about hearing loss and ways its impact can be lessened. There is also a fact sheet and other useful subsections.

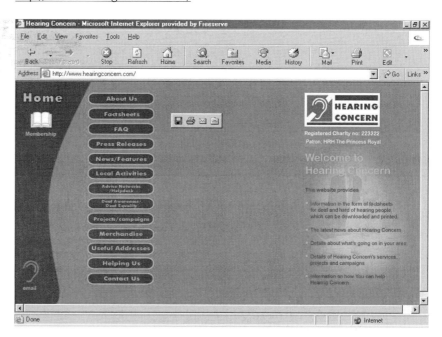

Ask NOAK: New York Online Access to Health
http://www.noah-health.org/

Here you will find high-quality full-text health information. You will find answers to many questions on a variety of health topics and resources. This site has received several awards.

BMJ
http://www.bmj.com/bmj/bmjpubs/sites.htm

This is a selection of WWW sites of medical interest.

Cancer Guide by a Recovered Cancer Patient
http://cancerguide.org

This is a guide put together by Steve Dunn who survived a diagnosis of cancer. He hopes his guide will help others.

Cancer OncoLink

http://cancer.med.upenn.edu

This site provides information on the many different types of cancer and the latest treatments. Topics include: psychosocial support, cancer causes and screening, clinical trials, frequently asked questions on cancer, and financial issues for cancer patients.

CANCERHELP

http://medweb.bham.ac.uk/cancerhelp/public.bacup

This is a free service about cancer and cancer care for the general public and health professionals. The site contains information for kids, adults and health professionals.

CancerWeb

http://www.graylab.ac.uk/cancerweb.html

This site offers information on cancer.

Centres for Disease Control and Prevention

http://www.cdc.gov

At this site you can read about prevention strategies for various diseases. You can even get more into the details with the scientific data, surveillance information, and health statistics. Also children by choice.

CYBERNURSE

http://www.cybernurse.com/

If you have an interest in being a nurse or have already taken the plunge, you should find this site useful.

Diabetes UK

http://www.diabetic.org.uk/

This site makes the point that over 1.4 million people in the UK have diabetes and another million probably have the condition but don't know it. This site brings together in one place information for people with diabetes. It is full of clearly stated facts and advice. Explanations about insulin, the pancreas, dietary needs, hypoglycaemia and other related subject are given.

Emergency Nursing on the Internet

http://www.Emergency-Nurse.com

The Accident and Emergency – Online has now been re-launched and is the home of A&E nursing on the Internet. Here you can search a selection of databases such as Medline, Toxline, Aidsline and Cancerlit. The databases are offered free of charge and no password or username is required to enter the site. New features include: Course and Conference calender, an articles and abstracts section, and more nursing humour. The existing sections have been improved and updated. There are now over 150 Emergency Nursing contacts in the e-directory, details on UK pay scales, information on the new UK nursing newsgroup 'uk-sci.med.nursing', and lots more.

Explore the Virtual Heart
http://sln.fi.edu/biosci/

At this site you will learn how a drug-free lifestyle helps your heart, exercise helps your heart, healthy eating helps your heart, you and your doctor can monitor your heart.
Reproduced by courtesy of The Franklin Institute Science Museum.

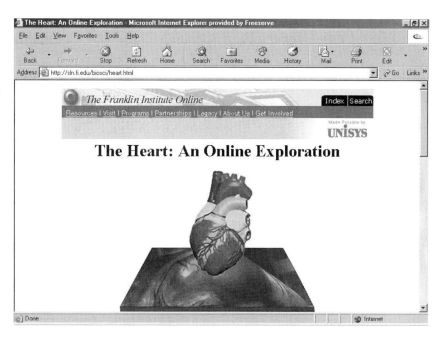

First Aid Sites
http://www.healing-aid.com/links.html
You can consult this site for health care advice on emergency situations. Links include: emergency medicine and primary care homepage, what to do during life-threatening emergencies, injury control resource information network, and National Collegiate EMS Foundation Home Page.

Healthcast
http://www.nbc12.com/healthcast/index.shtml
Here you will find various interesting stories and reports on a variety of health issues.

Hepatitis Network
http://www.hepnet.com/
This is an excellent site. It has an interactive learning section that is quite easy to use. It will update you on almost everything you need to know about hepatitis. It also has a 'Quick Search' option.

Medical On-line
http://www.medicalonline.com.au/
This site is home to a comprehensive array of information and access to major areas of medical interest. The site is designed to put both health professionals and the general public in contact with medical information.

Medical/Health Sciences Libraries on the web
http://www.arcade.uiowa.edu/hardin-www/hslibs.html
At this site you will find a meta-index of medical libraries that is organized by state and countries.

Medweb: Medical Libraries
http://www.MedWeb.Emory.edu/MedWeb

MedWeb is a catalogue of biomedical and health related web sites maintained by the staff of the Robert W. Woodruff Health Sciences Center Library at Emory University. Although MedWeb's primary audience is the academic and research community at Emory, you should find it equally useful. This site contains a list of almost 100 links to medical libraries.

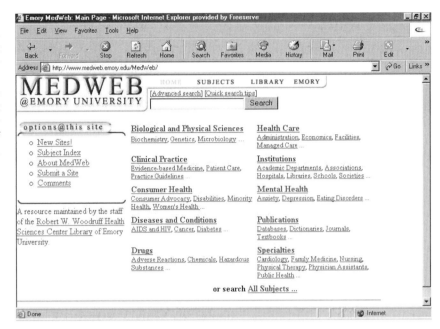

Medicines Homepage
http://www.pitt.edu/~cbw/altm.html

Therapies here can be classified as unconventional or innovative. Links include information on the following topics: acupuncture, chiropractic, Chinese medicine, medicinal herbs, osteopathic medicine, Chi, botanical medicine and many other general alternative medicine resources.

OMNI Gateway
http://omni.ac.uk

Outline medical networked information gateway for the UK.

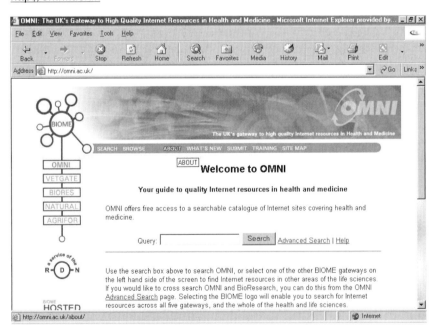

RX List

http://www.rxlist.com/

The Internet drug index. Search for a drug name or pull up the top 200 drugs by brand name, manufacturer and generic name.

Spina Bifida and Hydrocephalus

http://www.asbah.org

Here you will find comprehensive information on spina bifida. There are also links to other related sites.

The Virtual Medical Centre

http://sun2.lib.uci.edu/HSG/Medical.html

Although this site is primarily aimed at medical students, nursing and allied students would also find it beneficial. It has pages with detailed information in many different areas such as: endocrinology, haematology, ophthalmology, orthopaedics, urology and virology.

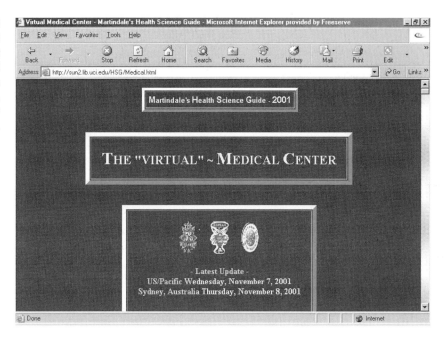

The Nutrition Expert

http://www.alaska.net/~tne/

This site provides information on the following: cholesterol, diabetes control, eating disorders, health food, sports nutrition, and weight loss.

Lab Tests

http://www.labtestsonline.org

This site is designed to help both patients and caregivers. Explanations are given on the tests patients are likely to undergo when they visit their doctor and the reason behind them. You will find a list describing why a test is given and how results are interpreted. Also available is a list of conditions and related tests. There are several in-depth articles covering areas such as anxiety during testing and reliability of home tests.

The Visible Human Project
http://www.nlm.nih.gov/research/visible/visible_human.html

Complete, anatomically detailed, three-dimensional representations of the male and female human body. Transverse CT, MRI and cryosection images of representative cadavers at one millimetre intervals.

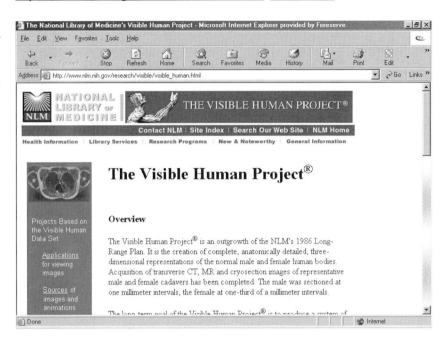

child nursing and medicine

Parenting/Child Health Information Database
http://www.cyh.com

This is a really useful site for people working in child health. It has 150 topics about childhood diseases, behaviour and parenting that can easily be printed out and given to parents.

Birth Defects Foundation
www.birthdefects.co.uk

The Birth Defects Foundation offers advice and support for parents whose children are born with a disease, syndrome or other kind of medical problem. Looking at research into birth defects and the support needed by parents, the site has a concise and informative style. You can find out about different conditions and also about national statistics for each kind of condition. This site is worth going to just to be aware of how much support is needed and provided for these parents.

Paediatric Points of Interest
http://www.med.jhu.edu/peds/neonatology/

Here you will find a searchable collection of links to resources in Paediatrics and Child health.

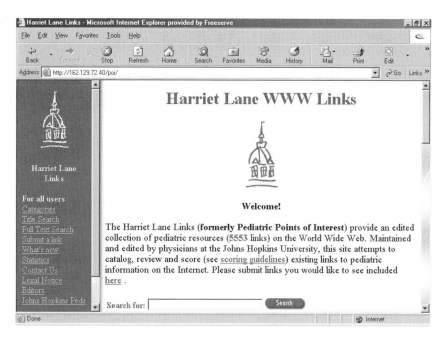

UK Parents
www.ukparents.co.uk

Not only an online community site, with the usual chat rooms and forums, UK Parents provides an opportunity to meet visitors at specially arranged coffee mornings across the country. The site aims to arm parents with health and developmental information about the challenges involved in bringing up young children, from troublesome teething to tantrum-throwing toddlers. There's a buy and sell facility, loads of stories and experiences and some fascinating new products, like the child finger protector, stopping children's fingers getting trapped.

learning disabilities

Disability Net
http://www.disabilitynet.co.uk

Disability Net is described by Paul Matthews as one of the world's leading Internet-based disability information and news services. The site contains a wide variety of information and offers many additional services such as Job Centre (if you are looking for a change in career) and Research (for requesting help with research projects, whether formal or informal).

ARC
http://TheArc.org

The Arc (formerly the Association for Retarded Citizens of the United States) is US's largest voluntary organization supported by contributions from the general public. The Arc comprises of individuals with mental retardation, family members, professionals in the field of disability and other concerned citizens. It has sections like government reports, questions and answers, discussion board and more.

The British Institute of Learning Disabilities
http://www.bild.org.uk/

At this site you will find a wide range of information related to learning disability. There is also a section on useful web links, which is quite extensive.

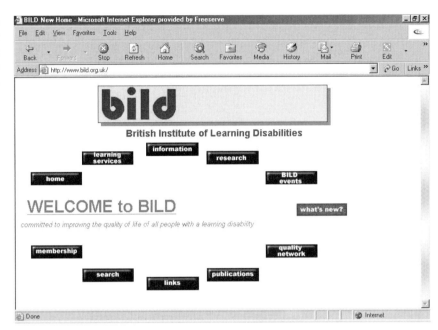

LD links
http://www.rnld.co.uk

This site is an excellent resource and provides a comprehensive listing of the current active web sites addressing the issues relevant to people with learning difficulties.

Learning Disabilities UK
http://www.learningdisabilitiesuk.org.uk

This site is by choice support and offers a number of resources related to current issues in learning disability care. The site also provides a comprehensive link-section to other relevant sites.

National Electronic Library for Health Learning Disabilities
http://minerva.minervation.com/ld

This site is a virtual branch library of the National Electronic Library for health and aims to provide access to the best current knowledge in relation to the development and delivery of services for people with learning disability.

mental health nursing and psychiatry

Department of Health – Mental Health
http://www.doh.gov.uk/mentalhealth

This is an excellent site containing all sorts of information for anyone with an interest in mental health nursing. Here you will find information relating to 'Mental Health Act 1983 and Human Rights'; the 'Five-Year Report of the National Confidential Inquiry into Suicide and Homicide by People with Mental Illness'; 'Making it Happen – A Guide to Delivering Mental Health Promotion', and much more.

Centre for Cognitive Therapy
http://hope4ocd.com
This California centre specializes in the treatment of obsessive-compulsive disorder using cognitive therapy methods. You will find Frequently Asked Questions (FAQ) and an online Y-BOCs Test.

Computers in Mental Health
http://www.ex.ac.uk/cimh/
This is a valuable site to visit. It contains a database of software and other resources.

Evidence-Based Mental Health On-line
http://www.ebmentalhealth.com/
This is a new full-text web site for EBMH launched in February 2001. It contains free sample issues. It has Searching and Browsing facilities. Using these facilities you can search or browse the archive of EBMH Online, which includes all issues of *Evidence Based Mental Health* published (the journal began in 1998). Full text (including figures and tables) and pdf files are available for issues published since February 1998.

Hyperguide to MHA 1983
http://www.hyperguide.co.uk/mha
At this site you will find a range of information related to the Mental Health Act 1983.

Internet Mental Health
http://www.mentalhealth.com/

This site is a free encyclopaedia of mental health issues. It contains information on the most common mental disorder, treatment and research. There is an online diagnostic program, which can used to diagnose Anxiety, Eating, Personality and Mood Disorders, Attention Deficiency Disorder, Schizophrenia and Substance-Related Disorders. Information on the most commonly prescribed psychiatric medicines is available.

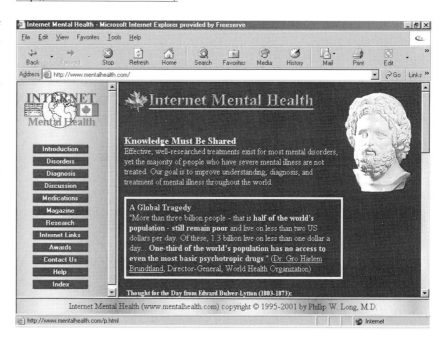

Institute of Psychiatry
http://www.iop.kcl.ac.uk/
This site, among other things, has a useful 'Student Forum' section. A click on this section will link you to BIDS, BioMedNet, a selection of online journals and more.

Mental Health Foundation
http://www.mentalhealth.org.uk/
This is the UK charity improving the lives of everyone with mental health problems or learning disabilities. At this site you will find links to various related sites.

The Samaritans
http://www.samaritans.org
This site offers a new way for the distressed and disturbed to get in touch. All e-mails are treated confidentially and there is a promise to give an answer within 24 hours. It also offers information on depression, the work of volunteers and how to offer support. You can also read reports, facts and figures on suicide in the UK.

eGuidelines
http://www.eguidelines.co.uk/
This site offers comprehensive information and practical solutions for clinical effectiveness. To get free access to eGuidelines you will need to complete an online registration form.

Centre for Evidence-based Mental Health
http://cebmh.com/
This site promotes and supports the teaching and practice of evidence-based mental health care. The Centre is a non-profit-making organization located within the University of Oxford Department of Psychiatry. At this site you can expect high-quality evidence-based mental health information, as well as a range of teaching materials.

Health of the Nation Outcome Scales (HoNOS)
http://www.honos.org.uk/index.htm
At this site you will be able to read about HoNOS, which is a 12-item Health of the Nation Outcome Scales developed by the UK Department of Health to measure the health and social functioning of people with severe mental illness. It contains 12 items measuring behaviour, impairment, symptoms and social functioning, and provides a means of recording progress towards the Health of the Nation target 'to improve significantly the health and social functioning of mentally ill people'. The scales were developed using stringent testing for acceptability, usability, sensitivity, reliability, and validity, and have been accepted by the NHS Executive Committee for Regulating Information Requirements for entry in the NHS Data Dictionary. The scales also form part of the Minimum Data Set for Mental Health.

midwifery and health visiting

Guide to Women's Health Issues
http://asa.ugl.lib.umich.edu/chdocs/womenhealth/toc.html
This site offers information on general health resources and emotional, physical and sexual health topics.

IVF and Infertility

www.ivf-infertility.co.uk

This is a site designed especially for people who are experiencing difficulty in having a child and think they may need medical help. You are taken through infertility causes, investigations and treatment options with clear and concisely written explanations. Latest research, such as the studying of every chromosome in an embryo to detect defects, and many other scientific breakthroughs are regularly posted.

Online Birth Centre

http://www.efn.org/~djz/birth/birthindex.html

Midwifery, pregnancy and birth-related information.

Pregnancy and Baby

www.ivillage.co.uk/pregnancyandbaby

This site has plenty on offer for parents or soon-to-be parents. Here you will find the latest developments in fertility treatments, contraception, birthing methods, and much more besides. Have some fun with the baby name finder, which will help you to choose a name for your new-born. You can also find out the origins and meaning of your name as well. Use the on-site expert sections to get helpful insights and advice.

Twins and Multiple Births Association

http://www.tamba.org.uk

This is a registered charity in the UK for all parents with twins, triplets, quads, quins, sextuplets or more. The site provides information and mutual support networks for families of twins or more.

Visible Embryo

http://www.visembryo.com/baby/index.html

This is an interesting site. You will be able to see the embryo at each stage of development and it also contains other materials including a quiz to keep you on your toes.

Women's Health Resources on the Internet

http://asa.ugl.lib.umich.edu:80/chdocs/womenhealth/womens_health.html

This site focuses on health issues that are of special interest to women and includes the following links: emotional health topics such as body image/eating disorders, relationships, and stress management; physical health issues such as fitness, nutrition and gynaecological exams; and sexual health issues such as pregnancy, the menopause and birth control.

Women's Health: Infertility

http://www.ferti.net/

This is a national awareness campaign site. It provides information on how to campaign and influence your MP, get more media coverage and set up a patient group. There are links to other sites.

BDA Dentistry
www.bda-dentistry.org.uk

This site is run by the British Dental Association. It is aimed at both the general public and also professionals. The site offers a handy 'find a dentist' service for you to locate your nearest surgery. There are informative articles on subjects such as whitening of teeth and taking up a career in dentistry, as well as a list of FAQs about dental work. You can read the list of facts and figures concerning the nation's teeth and also find out in detail about dental treatments. This helps to allay any fears you may have about certain procedures or operations.

Beyond Fear
www.beyondfear.org

This is another web site that aims to help those who are scared of the dentist deal appropriately with their phobia. It runs a registry of dentists who specialise in treating people suffering from dental fear. There are also helpful articles on methods of overcoming anxieties, different options available while in the dentist's chair, understanding the physiological effects of fear, and ways of preventing children from developing this fear of dentists. The self-help pages contain information on different pain relief methods (that don't involve a needle), and there are discussion groups for fellow sufferers.

Medical Education Software from other schools
http://www.med.virginia.edu/med-ed/otherMedEd.html

At this site you will find a listing of medical education software found at other schools, identified by category.

Information for Dentalphobics
http://www.dentalfear.org/

The page is written and published by Dr Stuart M. Ellis, Dental Surgeon, Cambridge, UK. There is a lot of information on dental phobia and how to deal with it.

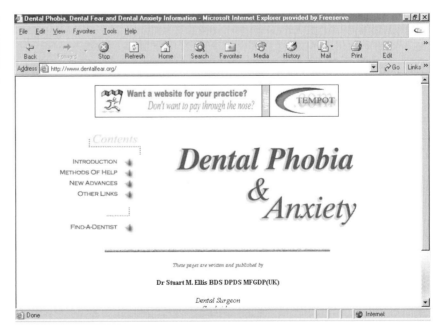

Virtual Reality in Medicine and Biology

http://www.shef.ac.uk/~vrmbg/

This site contains information on virtual reality in medicine and biology. Here you will find past and current research projects.

Medical Radiography Home Page

http://home.earthlink.net/~terrass/radiography/medradhome.html

The Medical Radiography Home Page provides a collection of links to Internet sites on a wide range of radiography topics. The resources are sorted into categories including physics, radiation protection, radiologic anatomy, education resources, medical imaging, medical informatics, general anatomy, radiology history, professional continuing education, professional organizations and societies, radiography software, study guides and practice tests, and other useful information sources.

Evidence-based Occupational Therapy

http://www.cebm.utoronto.ca/syllabi/occ/

This web site gives an introduction to evidence-based practice in occupational therapy. It is part of a series of resources developed and funded by the Center for Evidence-based Medicine at Mount Sinai Hospital in Toronto, Canada. The section on evidence-based occupational therapy includes an introduction to the key issues underlying evidence-based occupational therapy and a guide to other resources available to support education and practice.

complementary therapies

Acupuncture

http://www.medical-acupuncture.co.uk

This site is maintained by the British Medical Acupuncture Society. The site is packed with information for patients, practitioners and anyone with a passing interest. There is a list of the acupuncture specialists nearest to you and also a brief history of this ancient medical art. This is a great resource for a popular therapy.

Alternative Ways

www.alternativeways.co.uk

This guide to alternative treatment is run by Debbie Rye. She covers many areas of alternative therapy. At this site you can see what natural cures can do for problems such as asthma, backache, depression, and fatigue. Complete the online Lifestyle Analysis form to find out what areas you need to concentrate on, and send your results to Debbie for an even more in-depth appraisal by e-mail. Learn about invisible geopathic and electromagnetic stress, which apparently cause ill health.

Alexander Technique, the Complete Guide
http://www.alexandertechnique.com

This is a site that is well worth a visit. Here you will find a systematic guide to the Alexander Technique plus other resources – both on and off the Internet.

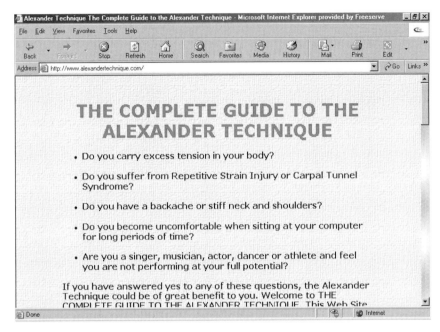

Aromatherapy
http://www.fragrant.demon.co.uk
This is a guide to aromatherapy and thousands of links, including 600 aromatherapy sites.

Beaumont College
www.beaumontcollege.co.uk
The interest in alternative therapies has grown beyond recognition in the past ten years. If you are interested in how to become a professional practitioner then Beaumont College could be the place for you. Under the tutelage of Denise Whichello Brown you can study massage, aromatherapy or reflexology. This internationally renowned lecturer on complementary medicine offers part-time, intensive and residential courses. You can read testimonials from other former students and find out where the courses are run and where to stay while you study.

Health Library
www.internethealthlibrary.com
The Health Library claims to be the largest source of alternative medicine, complementary therapy and natural health care resources in the UK. Going by what's on offer here they are probably right. Alongside the web store featuring hundreds of natural remedies there is a stress tester, a remedy finder and a large directory of clinics and practitioners. The latest news is kept well up to date and the University of Exeter's Department of Complementary Medicine supports all the material. A new practitioner search engine has just been added to the site.

Healthy Pages
www.healthypages.co.uk
If you're looking for an alternative or complementary method of treatment then this is the site to go to. Healthy Pages claims to be the UK's fastest growing

complementary health directory. It has information on all types of alternative therapists, from practitioners of acupressure to yoga teachers all over the country. Complementary health practitioners can advertise free here too. Packed with all the latest developments in the world of alternative health, the site is very soundly researched. You can also search for a clinic, a specialist in Reiki or whatever treatment you desire, near to you.

Inter Connections
www.interconnections.co.uk
This guide to holistic and preventative treatments concentrates on two main principles. The holistic approach to medicine recognizes that illnesses and overt symptoms are often evidence of underlying problems: emotional, mental or connected with lifestyle and attitude. The preventative medicine tries to bring about a positive state of health and well-being without treating actual symptoms. Feng shui, psychotherapy, meditation and shamanism are just a few of the therapies covered in this interesting site.

Therapy World
www.therapy-world.co.uk
If you are interested in stepping away from orthodox treatments and experimenting with alternative therapies then this is the place to go. There is a stack of information on all kinds of therapy and the site has a list of eight steps you should take in order to find the right therapist for you. Aromatherapy, hypnotherapy, nutritional therapy, and physiotherapy are just a few of the subjects covered. The links and lists of practitioners are very helpful and the descriptions of treatments are honest.

Think Natural
www.thinknatural.com
Are you looking for a natural way to ease the stresses and strains of modern living? Then visit this site. Think Natural is a UK-based site containing a huge amount of information on natural health therapies. There is an encyclopaedia from Dorling Kindersley, and contributions from specialist journalists and natural health practitioners on hundreds of different methods and remedies. Therapies, for example, include herbs and medicinal plants, minerals, Bach flower remedies, and aromatherapy. The core of the site is a well-stocked online shop selling everything from massage oils to St John's Wort. The Health File covers all aids and ailments, from aches and pains to stress and vitality.

health education

Feeling Fat
www.feelingfat.net
This Feeling Fat site has everything you need to be successful at slimming. There is a slimming shop with a variety of special offers on slimming aids and goods, slimming advice, online programmes, and diaries. You can record your weight loss on a progress chart and read countless slimming success stories to inspire those pounds to fall off! With special tips for men who need to lose weight, guides to exercising and suggestions for healthy breaks, this site has it all.

Giving Up Smoking

http://www.givingupsmoking.co.uk

Smoking is unarguably a filthy habit. If you have been looking for help to give up then you should find all the help you need at this site. It offers every kind of support and positive thinking. There are sections on why to give up, how to give up and how to stay stopped. You will also find advice how to persuade friends or family to give up as well, without nagging or badgering them.

Health World

http://www.health.net

At this site you will have the delight of travelling around a 'virtual health village' and gather a vast amount of information on almost every aspect of healthy living. It is easy to find whatever information you require. You can choose from Fitness Centre, Healthy Family, Health News, and Nutrition Centre, to name but a few of the categories. Once inside a category you can read all the latest news and search for particular topics. The information at this site is regularly updated.

Home Health

http://www.homehealth-uk.com

At this site you will find facts, theories and comments on every common ailment and disease you may contract. Test kits are available, ranging from a pregnancy test to blood tests for digestive disorders and diabetes, and urine tests for cystitis. New to the site is an online consultant who helps you to monitor your health from home.

Mind Body Soul

http://www.mindbodysoul.gov.uk

This site is divided into sections covering a range of different health topics. Examples of topics covered are: accidents, alcohol, drugs, healthy eating, mental health, physical activity, sexual health, smoking, and sun safety. The health conditions section is excellent and contains expert explanations and descriptions of different medical conditions. Each section is packed with facts, figures and useful advice. There are also plenty of links to other sites dealing with issues presented on the links page. A useful site for anyone and any age.

Nutrition

http://www.nutrition.org.uk

This site is run by the British Nutrition Foundation (BNF). It contains excellent articles and advice on how to eat more healthily. You can study the nutrition of facts, read about all the latest news and research, and even find out about hygiene and food safety. The BNF shows how it is trying to instil healthy eating by educating younger and older generations and also how it can help students with information on Food Technology courses.

Healthy Living Exercise Zone
www.funtime.demon.co.uk

If you believe that 'an ounce of effort is worth a ton of theory' then this is a site for you. So when you can muster up that spare ounce of energy to do some exercise instead of wasting it on fruitless theoretical talk, go to this site. There you will find exercise routines to work out every muscle group and help build up your stamina, strength, speed, or whatever area you want. There are different routines for your fitness level and the exercises are clearly described. A simple site with easy-to-follow instructions and good sports science.

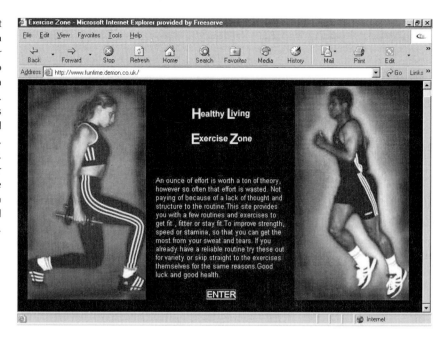

Surgery Door
http://www.surgerydoor.co.uk

This is a great online resource. You will find a whole range of information and advice pertaining to hundreds of different topics – bad breath, blood clots, migraines, and cancer to name but a few. There are pages here for women's health, men's health, complementary medicine, health for the over 50s, and much, much more. A huge authoritative site packed with handy links.

Web MD
http://www.msn.co.uk/health

This site contains a collection of articles, tips and advice on both physical and emotional matters. The illustrated guides are very informative and provide clear explanations of many health issue and conditions.

health care research

Research & Development Co-ordinating Centre
http://www.man.ac.uk/rcn

The web site has been developed to provide an easy-to-access means of sharing information on research and practice development in nursing, and is designed to be fully interactive.

The Cochrane Collaboration
http://www.cochrane.org/

The Cochrane Collaboration is an international not-for-profit organization. At this site you should find up-to-date, accurate information about the effects of health care. Reviews are prepared mostly by health care professionals who volunteer to work in one of the more than 40 Collaborative Review Groups. Also pay a visit to: http://cochrane.mcmaster.ca/

Digest of Health-Related Research Funding and Training Opportunities
http://www.rdinfo.org.uk/

Here you will find a selected list of major funding sources. The list is regularly updated and contains those sources that are most likely to be relevant.

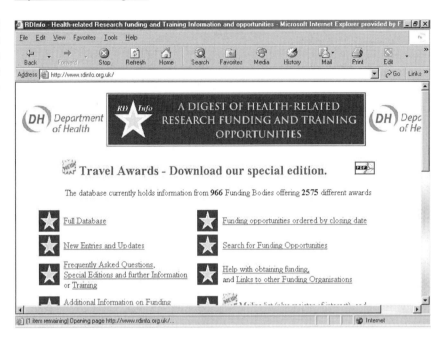

journals for health professionals

British Journal of Community Health Nursing
http://www.britishjournalofcommunitynursing.com/
A peer-reviewed monthly community nursing journal, promoting excellence in primary care. The journal is primarily of interest to district nurses, health visitors, school nurses, and community psychiatric nurses. In addition to clinical reviews and editorials, features include professional updates, innovations in practice, research and development, policy and practice as well as specialist, in-depth supplements on each issue.

British Journal of Health Care Management
http://www.bjhcm.com/
The British Journal of Health Care Management was founded in 1995, with the remit to examine the big ideas, issues and debates in managing health care for the twenty-first century, looking at the lessons, the reality, the theories, the politics, and the practice. It is a monthly publication, aiming at managers in health care organizations, and combines peer reviewed-papers and the articles with top-level columnists. You can access on-line a selection of articles from the print edition. These are updated monthly for you to keep ahead on the latest news and views in health care management.

British Journal of Midwifery
http://www.britishjournalofmidwifery.com/
British Journal of Midwifery is the leading clinical peer-reviewed journal for midwives. Its strong readership is an indication of the winning combination of quality clinical content and in-depth clinical supplements. The *BJM* meets the growing demand to provide the latest clinical and educational information needed to succeed in midwifery.

British Journal of Therapy and Rehabilitation
http://www.bjtr.co.uk/
Welcome to BJTR.co.uk, the world's only multidisciplinary web site for therapist and rehabilitation professionals. BJTR.co.uk's aim is to act as an online resource for all rehabilitation professionals in the UK and abroad.

Evidence-Based Nursing
http://www.bmjpg.com/
Evidence-Based Nursing is a new high-quality international journal. This journal gives you access to the best research related to nursing and keeps you up to date with the most important new evidence in nursing. What's more, *Evidence-Based Nursing* help you to put this evidence into practice, as expert commentators put every article into a clinical context and draw out the key research findings. Every edition of *Evidence-Based Nursing* contains 24 different summaries covering a wide variety of nursing-related issues which are relevant to you. This journal is published by BMJ Publishing Group, a commercial division of the British Medical Association (BMA).

British Journal of Nursing
http://www.britishjournalofnursing.com/

The clinical review journal for nurses with an emphasis on education and debate. *BJN* is peer-reviewed and refereed, which is an essential requirement for a journal of authority. The journal contains regular additional supplements on children's nursing, learning disabilities, adult/elderly care, mental health, and specialist nursing. The clinical section covers all subjects and issues relating to clinical practice. Other subjects include surgical nursing, the wound care clinic, ethical and legal issues, research, and management.

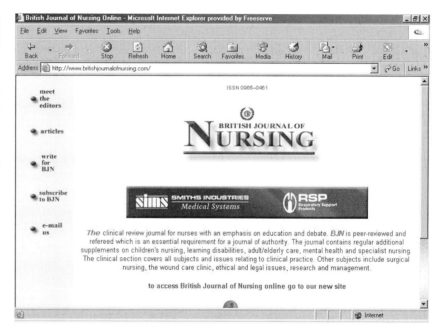

Health Service Journal (HSJ)
http://www.hsj.co.uk
The HSJ online is the UK's leading health policy and management web site. It is the interactive version of the *Health Service Journal*. It has an average of 100,000 page impressions per week. At present the information provided on HSJ online is free. Recently included is a section called HSJ Jobs Plus, which carries all job adverts that have appeared in the *Health Service Journal*. You can search for jobs according to category and location, and respond immediately via e-mail. HSJ Jobs Plus also includes an extensive training section and details of the latest NHS tenders.

UNIVERSITY OF HERTFORDSHIRE LRC

Health Informatics Journals
http://www.shef.ac.uk/uni/projects/hij

This is an international journal for any health care professional involved with information, information technology and computing. It has an impressive editorial team with Chris Dowd as Executive editor. It aims to emphasize the central role of information and the application of information technology in clinical practice, by ensuring that papers which are practice-based are actively encouraged and assisted to publication. All papers are subjected to a full review process by experts in the relevant field. The journal has four issues per year.

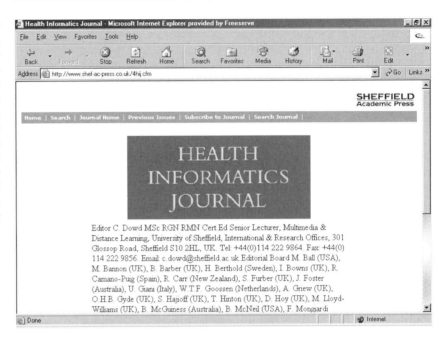

Hospital Medicine
http://www.hospitalmedicine.co.uk/

Hospital Medicine is an international, peer-reviewed clinical review journal. It covers all hospital specialties, as reflected by its Editorial Board and International Advisory Board. It contains review articles written by experts in each field, allowing busy doctors quickly and easily to update their knowledge on a particular area. *Hospital Medicine* was launched in 1966 and since then has constantly provided doctors with an independent source of clinical information in an easily digestible format. Each issue contains editorials, a symposium or three or four articles on one particular topic, review articles, education and training updates, looking at issues affecting both the trainee and the trainer, case reports, correspondence, and book reviews.

International Journal of Palliative Nursing
http://www.internationaljournalofpalliativenursing.com/

International Journal of Palliative Nursing has developed into a major force for this rapidly growing speciality. It has gained respect and credibility for providing palliative nurses throughout the world with a high-quality, peer-reviewed journal. It has become the 'bible' for palliative nurses wishing to stay ahead in this demanding and rapidly growing speciality. The *IJPN* is peer-reviewed and refereed with regular sections on nursing innovations, symptom management, education, and international developments.

Practice Nursing
http://www.practicenursing.com/

A fortnightly for nurses and managers working in general practice, with a heavy emphasis on quality clinical articles which are required by the practice team to update their skills. Its professional approach updates nurses and managers with clinical reviews, clinical supplements and educational articles. The information in the popular walk-in clinic is a useful feature for revision purposes, providing a full check list on the management and treatment of each condition.

RCN Nursing Standard Online

http://www.nursing-standard.co.uk

At this web site you will find a selection of articles and abstracts from the weekly issue of *Nursing Standard*, plus details of conferences and continuing education opportunities.

Nursing and Residential Care

http://www.nursingresidentialcare.com/

A first-class journal for the professional and clinical needs of care assistants, care workers, nurses, residential care workers and managers working in both nursing and residential care homes. This peer-reviewed journal includes up-to-date clinical reviews, self-directed learning, professional issues, regular product focuses and jobs and courses.

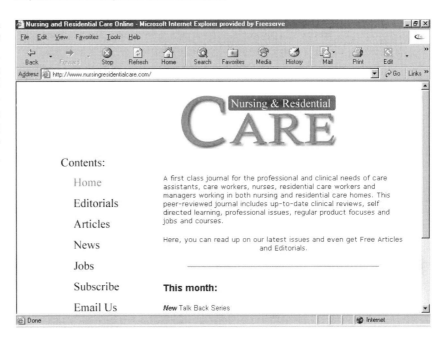

British Medical Journal online

http://www.bmj.com

The *BMJ* contains many traditional paper-based articles. It provides free full-text articles and it is fully searchable. Note that although the *BMJ* is freely available, most electronic journals charge a subscription fee and require a password in order to gain full-text access.

libraries and free health care databases

AIDS Information Service

http://www.oneworld.net/

The One World database contains tens of thousands of documents on AIDS.

ENB Health Care Database Search

http://enb-search.ulcc.ac.uk/cgi-bin/hcdsearch

This is a bibliographical database with abstracts for each entry. That is, it acts as a signpost to journal articles and research reports but does not store the full text. You will need to ask at your library for the original sources – journals or reports. If they are not held in stock, your library should be able to order them for you through the British Library's inter-library loan system. As at March 2002, the Database contains nearly 58,000 records from UK health care journals since 1986. It also contains information about health care organizations and about open-learning course providers.

Healthworks Online: Health and Medical Information Service

http://www.healthworks.co.uk

A UK information service. Here you will have free access to Medline from home, college or any Internet-connected PC with unlimited searches.

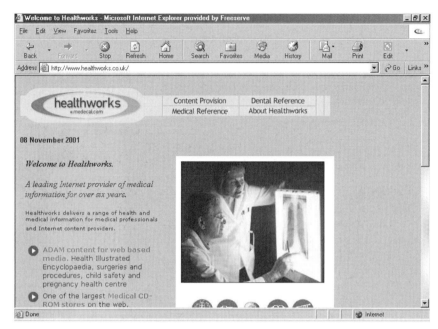

HENSA

http://www.hensa.ac.uk

This is a national service that benefits the higher education and research community in the UK. It maintains copies of electronic archives from all over the world, providing access to a wide range of up-to-date software and other material that is available free of charge to anyone from the UK HE community.

Interactive Patient Home Page

http://medicus.marshall.edu/medicus.htm

Test your diagnostic skills. *The Interactive Patient* at Marshall University School of Medicine is a truly unique interactive World Wide Web program that allows the user to simulate an actual patient encounter. This teaching tool for physicians, residents and medical students offers a case with a chief complaint to the user, who then has to interact with the patient requesting additional history, performing a physical exam, and reviewing laboratory data and x-rays. After the workup, the user is encouraged to submit a diagnosis and a treatment plan to the system based on the information obtained. All submitted answers are evaluated and feedback is provided.

Internet Public Library

http://www.ipl.org

This is the first public library of and for the Internet community. When you visit this site you will find a useful section called FAQs where you will find the answers to all your questions about this site.

MUSC – Occupational Therapy Home

http://www.musc.edu/chp-rehab/ot/othome.htm

This page is being developed as a comprehensive resource for information regarding the MUSC program, events relating to OT in South Carolina, and resources that would be valuable to occupational therapists everywhere.

NHS Direct Online

http://www.nhsdirect.nhs.uk

At this site you will find reliable and knowledgeable diagnosis. Simply click on the relevant part of the body key, answer 'yes' or 'no' to the subsequent questions, and you'll be told whether you should wait till the local health centre opens, call out the doctor, or ring 999.

National Electronic Library for Health (NeLH)

http://www.nelh.nhs.uk

This is a pilot site which aims to provide clinicians with access to the best current know-how and knowledge to support health-care related decisions. All content on this site is free. The majority of information can be accessed by all users. But some of the content is restricted to certain users, who will need to register for a password in order to use them. It also provides useful links to relevant databases. Patients, carers and the public too can use this site, but they might find NHS Direct Online (see above) a better gateway for health information.

Open Software Library (OSL)

http://www.personal.u-net.com/~osl/

OSL publishes and distributes education and training material for nurses and other health professionals. Here you will find software on CD-ROMs, disks and videos covering a wide spectrum of nursing and health care education.

Virtual Hospital HomePage – University of Iowa

http://vh.org

The Virtual Hospital is a digital health sciences library created in 1992 at the University of Iowa to help meet the information needs of health care providers and patients. The goal of the Virtual Hospital digital library is to make the Internet a useful medical reference and health promotion tool for health care providers and patients. It contains hundreds of books and brochures for health care providers and patients.

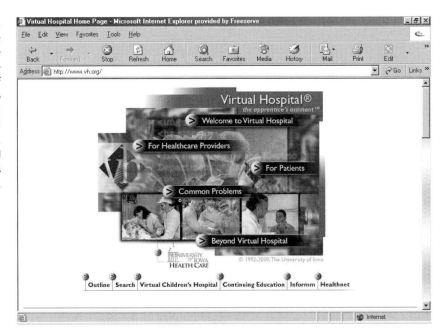

Resources for Nurses and Families

http://pegasus.cc.ucf.edu/~wink/home.html

Here is a site where you will find teaching resources, Internet search engines, Internet resources, and much more.

organizations, associations and uk statutory bodies

All Cures

http://www.allcures.com

This is a UK-based web site. It offers products that you will normally expect to find in any high-street pharmacy. You can also get detailed advice if you use the 'ask the pharmacist' section, and there is a link to Netdoctor.co.uk, for health care advice.

Alzheimer's Association

http://www.alzheimers.org.uk

This site contains links to other resources and information on chapter contacts, conferences and events, and medicine and caregivers.

Arthritis and Rheumatism Council

http://rheuma.bham.ac.uk/arc.html

This is a major UK charity dedicated to supporting research and education relating to joint diseases. The web site has a range of information for patients, health care professionals and researchers.

British Computer Society Nursing Specialist Group

http://www.bcsnsg.org.uk/

This nursing specialist group is one of five Health Informatics Specialist Groups of the British Computer Society and contributes to the national and international debates on information management and technology issues within health care. At this site you will find information on all the focus groups.

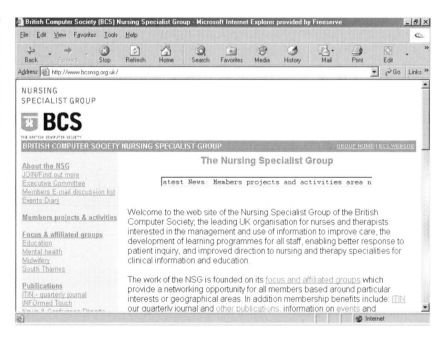

British Digestive Foundation

http://www.bdf.org.uk/

This is the only national charity that is concerned with all forms of digestive disorders. The site provides information for sufferers, their families and friends.

British Epilepsy Association

http://www.epilepsy.org.uk/

Here you will find all sorts of information on epilepsy. Information is organized under the following sections: a parents' guide to epilepsy; employment; self-management; women; medical management; leisure; education; driving.

British Heart Foundation (BHF)

http://www.bhf.org.uk

The BHF, established in 1961, plays an essential part in funding heart research in the UK. This site gives you information on how they fund the research, what research is being carried out and how it helps to reduce the ever-present problem of heart disease. Also available at this site are the latest news on heart disease and what medical terms regarding the heart mean.

Natural Oils Research Association Site

http://www.acemake.com/NORA/

A very interesting site to visit.

Department of Health (DoH)

http://www.open.gov.uk/doh/dhhome.htm

Homepage of the government department. It has details of, among other things, the Health of the Nation plus updates and research findings.

Information for Health

http://www.nhsia.nhs.uk

At this site you will find information about government policy with regards to IT in a modern NHS. A description of how electronic patient and health records will be developed to support the health care process is given; the infrastructure that must be in place to support local action is identified; what must be done to improve the flow and use of information for health improvement, clinical governance, performance management and national service frameworks is addressed; how the information needs of patients and the general public will be met is also addressed; what needs to happen at national and local levels is outlined; and the scene for detailed implementation guidance by discussing resources and local implementation timescales is set.

Screenshot reproduced with the permission of the NHS Information Authority.

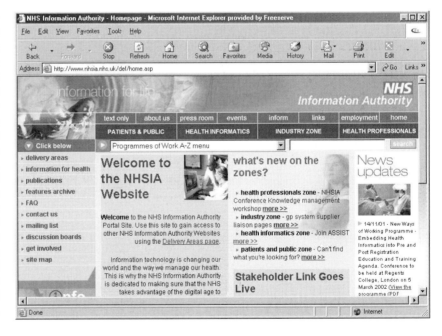

Marie Stopes Institute

http://www.mariestopes.org.uk/

This site provides all sorts of information relating to people's right to have children by choice.

Multiple Sclerosis Society

http://www.mssociety.org.uk/

This society supports people whose lives are affected by multiple sclerosis by funding research and provides local and national services. At this site you will find information on drug therapies, welfare publications and information for professionals. There is also a Frequently Asked Questions (FAQ) section.

NAHAT (National Association of Health Authorities and Trusts)

http://www.doh.gov.uk

Here you will find the latest on the Department's work, as well as health and social care guidance, publications and policies.

National Board of Nursing, Midwifery and HV in Scotland

http://www.nbs.org.uk

This site is similar to its sister site – the English National Board. It contains various regulations and guidelines, the board publications and so on.

Netdoctor

http://www.netdoctor.co.uk

This is an excellent reference site. The interactive sections are well put together. You can test yourself or ask Dr Hilary Jones a question in his live surgery session, which takes place every Monday. If you submit your query 30 minutes before the surgery starts you should receive an answer. You will also find a useful directory of all your local health centres with contact details.

NMC (Nursing and Midwifery Council)

http://www.nmc-uk.org/

On 1 April 2002, the United Kingdom Central Council (UKCC) was replaced by another body called the Nursing and Midwifery Council (NMC). This council was set up by Parliament to ensure nurses, midwives and health visitors provide high standards of care to their patients and clients. At this web site you will find information about the NMC and its activities.

Online Medical

http://www.medical-library.org

This site was created by the National Medical Society. Here visitors will have an assessment of their symptoms with a program created by 1,500 specialist physicians. It generates a diagnosis based upon your condition and includes treatment options for over 1,200 diseases. This is a well-prepared and well-resourced site.

Prostate Help Association

http://www.u-net.com/~pha/

This is a registered charity. The site offers information on all types of prostate disease.

Royal College of Nursing (RCN)
http://www.thebiz.co.uk

Human resources, training and development, membership and other information.

World Health Organization (WHO)
http://www.who.int

This site continues to be a must-visit for any health care professionals and students of health studies who are interested about the state of health worldwide. There are reams of detailed and far-reaching aspect of world health. At this site you can view issues currently under discussion, from the outbreak and spread of diseases such as malaria to the success stories of health education and programmes in developing countries. Other sections include environment, health technology and new UN policy.

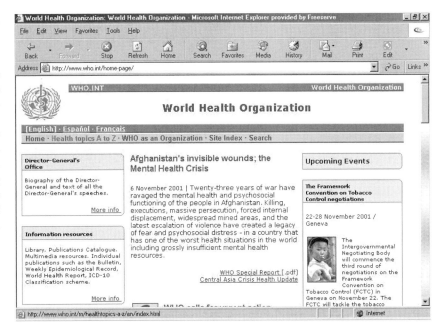

---

electronic publications and citations

Internet Publishing
http://www.sscnet.ucla.edu/ssc/franks/book

This is the HTML version of the *Internet Publishing Handbook for World-Wide Web, Gopher, and WAIS* by Mike Franks. It is complete with publication data, a collection of Internet links (URLs) from the book, and a note on differences between the HTML and printed versions of this book. The paper version is available in bookstores.

Untangling the Web

http://www.eeicommunications.com/eye/utw/

This is a column about the Internet, especially World Wide Web publishing. It appears here on this web site every month as well as on the newsletter at this web site: http://www.eeicommunications.com/eye/

At this site, you are alerted to useful and interesting resources on the Internet. Confusing terms are defined. Myths are debunked. You can also find loads of tips on writing and designing a web site.

(For additional help refer to Unit 9 in this book.)

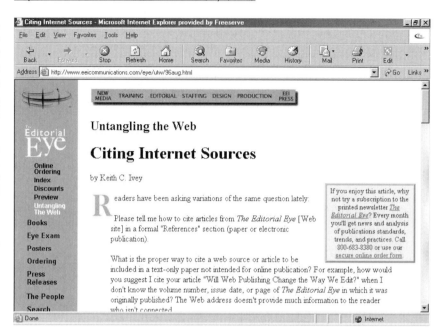

I hope you have managed to access all the sites listed above and you have found some, if not all, of them useful. Some web sites are updated more often than others. New ones are appearing all the time, while others vanish into thin air. As you get attached to the net you will discover new sites.

summary and conclusion

With the help of a suitable browser such as Internet Explorer or NetScape Navigator/Communicator you can surf through the net jumping from place to place in computer databases all over the world by using the hypertext links. You can also browse the net by using URLs you know about, or try the ones listed in this Unit. Do remember that the net is constantly changing. Therefore when you encounter an address to which you cannot connect, try connecting to the host system without specifying a specific document. For example, suppose you have typed this URL:

http://www.sscnet.ucla.edu/ssc/franks/book

. . . and you cannot connect, then try:

http://www.sscnet.ucla.edu/

unit 4
finding health information on the internet

Trained as a librarian, I find the web untidy. Libraries are organized according to established principles, and if you understand them, you can find your way around any library. The Web has protocols for data transfer, but beyond that, there's inconsistency

(Lane, 1996)[6]

Searching the Internet for specific information is a daunting prospect for most of us, rather like being presented with the task of finding a very small fly in a very large web!

Howson (1997)[7]
Information Officer, ScHARR – University of Sheffield
Email n.j.howson@sheffield.ac.uk

Note It is important to remember that not all the material on the net is free. While there are many electronic journals available online, some of them require subscriptions before you can view the full text. Many databases are also offered as a fee-paying service. However, if your institution has a subscription to some of these journals and databases, you will be able to gain access at the college. If you would like to gain access from your home computer, see your librarian for help and advice.

The Internet increases in size daily. Uncalculable numbers of pages are added all over the world in every language and in every subject. With so much information in cyberspace, you may wonder where you should start to find and isolate the medical and health information you want. Wonder no more. There are some simple techniques and some wonderful people out there who have created sophisticated tools that you can use to make it easy for you to find what you are looking for. Once you develop some skill with them, the results will be gratifying. You will find what you need and maybe even discover something you didn't know you wanted.

Once upon a time, you could search for information on the net by 'surfing' and making educated guesses about which links to follow from a few selected web pages to find the information you needed. Unfortunately, the extraordinary growth of the Internet has rendered that strategy about as successful as looking for a lost needle in a haystack. You may enjoy the challenge, but you are unlikely to find what you need. To find your way around you need a plan of action. Taking time to think about what you want before you hop on the net can save you a lot of time and effort.

In this unit you will be introduced to a few valuable tools that are ridiculously easy to use. You will get to meet some other inhabitants of the net: Web Directories, Search Engines, Information Gateways and Online Databases. You will also have an opportunity to explore specific databases using effective search strategies to make your searches both pleasant and successful.

Below is a checklist for what you can expect to find out in this unit. Read through the statements then tick (✓) the items about which you would like to know more.

I would like to find out more about:

Please now read through the topics you have ticked.

Web Directories or **Subject Trees** are hand-built lists of pages sorted into categories. Although you can search directories using a keyword search, it's often as easy to click on a category and then click your way through the ever-more specific subdirectories until you find the subject you're interested in. The downside is that they won't always find the newest sites. Sites get listed in directories when their authors submit them for inclusion. (See Section 4.1.2.)

Search Engines are databases containing indexes of WWW sites built automatically by a program called a spider, a robot, a crawler, or a worm. These programs constantly visit the web and return with information about a page's location, titles and contents, which is then added to an index (a searchable catalogue of web pages). Search engines have the benefit of being up to date but the downside is that if, for example, you search for viral meningitis, the resulting list won't necessarily contain information about meningitis of the viral type – some may just be pages in which the words 'viral' and 'meningitis' both happen to appear. (See Section 4.1.3.)

Information Gateways are similar to web directories. They can be viewed as an online catalogue. They have only details of the very best links in a particular subject. The process of filtering is carried out by a team of experts employed for that purpose. Some gateways specialize in particular subjects while others cover a range of subjects. (See Section 4.1.4.)

Most of the information you need for your important research project is probably out there – somewhere – online, and it is probably indexed or catalogued somehow. Unfortunately for us, the Internet wasn't set up by librarians who organize things in a logical way and provide a central index to make them easy to find. We should not let this discourage us from accessing the millions of web pages in cyberspace, because among them lies valuable information on all aspects of health.

Although there is no one right way to search the net for information, there are, however, two main methods of information seeking online. They are:

- **Browsing** – this involves moving from one website to another, following links that you think might lead you to the information you need, or
- **Searching** – which involves putting key words or phrases in a search box.

To carry out an effective search, there are also several valuable tools you can use and techniques you can develop to refine your searches. **Web Directories**, **Search Engines** and **Information Gateways** (also called Subject Gateways) are three valuable tools that will help you find materials on the web. They are designed to help you navigate the Internet quickly and efficiently. There are various species of the Web Directories, Search Engines and Information Gateways. The number is growing all the time.

Starting pages are web pages. They provide you with a useful set of hyperlinks to general reference information. All you need to do is to survey the list of topics and choose a link that interests you. No search skills or strategies are needed.

If you are using the computer lab in your college or university, you may find that when you access the Internet the homepage may contain links to information you need, such as e-mail addresses of your colleagues, Web Search and Links, Hot Links to popular pages and so on. On the other hand, if you are accessing the net on your home computer, you will most likely get the homepage of your ISP (Internet Service Provider). The homepage usually provides you with useful links to explore. But for students of health studies and health professionals there are more useful pages to start with.

4.1.1.1 the virtual library

If you are collecting information for a research project, then the library is usually one of the first places you go to. However, instead of visiting traditional libraries, you can use the net to visit one of several virtual libraries. One of them is in fact called 'The Virtual Library' and you will find it at: http://www.w3.org/vl/

4.1.1.2 reference desk

Always try to find tools that work most of the time, but be prepared to use others if you are not satisfied with the results.

This is the online equivalent of a library reference desk. The main page offers a set of choices, including reference tools, current news, help and advice, plus more. After choosing any of them, you will find even more links to explore. You can find the Reference Desk at: http://www.refdesk.com/index.html

Unlike Search Engines, most Web Directories are created by humans (rather than robots). Human editors select and organize the web pages into various categories, sometimes with reviews and ratings of web sites. However, there are a few Web Directories that are partly automated: resources are found by a piece of software and are then arranged into categories by a human editor. In both cases, resources are organized hierarchically and allow you to browse through a range of health subject areas that are arranged from the broad to the specific. In addition to browsing, Web Directories also allow you to search using search terms and key words. By and large, Web Directories will help you find the haystack and other tools will help you find the needle. Table 4.1 outlines five of the best.

Table 4.1	Yahoo!	http://www.yahoo.co.uk
Popular Web Directories	**UK & Ireland**	Yahoo! has been around since 1994. According to recent evaluations and studies, Yahoo! is the best subject tree to start with and one that has consistently been found to be both useful and fun. It is a searchable, browsable hierarchical index of the Internet. Yahoo! highlights listings that are about or are of particular interest to web users in the UK, Ireland and the expatriate community. Its coverage is general, but searching and browsing can be limited to health topics.
	Achoo	http://www.achoo.com/ This is a health focus version of Yahoo covering approximately 7,000 indexed and searchable sites. It has three main categories: practice of medicine, human life and the business of health. Although there is a searching facility, browsing the index is a better option. An updated and improved version is under development, to include better searching facilities.
	BUBL Link	To access this site you must type the keyword: **BUBL Link** in the Address box of your browser. BUBL LINK is the name of a catalogue of selected Internet resources covering all academic subject areas and catalogued according to DDC (Dewey Decimal Classification). All items are selected, evaluated, catalogued, and described. Links are checked and fixed each month. LINK stands for Libraries of Networked Knowledge. The BUBL LINK catalogue currently holds over 11,000 resources. This is far smaller than the databases held by major search engines, but it can provide a more effective route to information for many subjects, across all disciplines.
	InfoSeek Select Sites	http://guide.infoseek.com/ This directory has several categories including Health and Medicine.
	Magellan	http://www.mckinley.com/ This directory includes categories such as Communications, Daily Living, Food, Health, Humanities, Science, Law, Environment, and Spirituality. This is another subject index, which can be searched by keyword. What makes it different, however, is that it provides both ratings and reviews for sites you find through its subject index. If you do a keyword search instead, it will also provide a brief description of the sites that come up. These reviews and ratings are quite useful in determining whether the sites are worth exploring.

4.1.2.1 carrying out a search using a web directory

Most search tools tend to be biased towards the US. It may be worthwhile to start our first activity in this section with a tool that is very easy to use and that allows us to limit to just the UK. For this reason I have picked Yahoo! – but it is important to bear in mind that most web directories work in the same way, and also look much the same.

Activity 4.1 making a simple search using yahoo!

Suppose we wanted to find some information on a particular medical condition, let's say *Meningitis*. We can ask Yahoo! to use this keyword to search its entire database and offer a list of sites containing information on this medical condition.

For hands-on experience, carry out the steps listed in **Worksheet 5**.

When you are done, please return to this page and read on.

Worksheet 5 searching with yahoo!'s web directory

 Note When you arrive at the Yahoo! site you will see a page like the one shown in the screenshot. You will notice it has a search-engine style textbox into which you can type keywords. Since we know exactly what we are looking for (i.e. information on meningitis), we can use this textbox to do a search.

1 Log on to Windows.
2 Start your browser.
3 Enter the following URL in the location/address box:

http://www.yahoo.co.uk

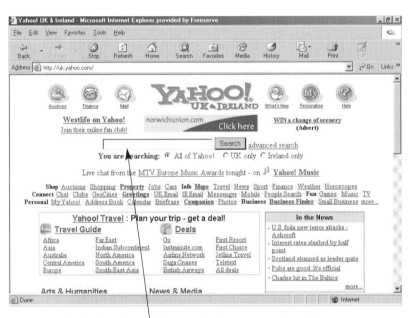

4 Point and click in this textbox. *A flashing cursor should appear.*
5 Type the keyword: **meningitis**, then click the **Search** button. *After a few seconds you should see a new page listing the sites that matched your search criteria.*
6 Click on any of the links that interest you. If the page does not interest you, click on the **Back** button on your browser's toolbar to return to the search results and try a different one. When you have had enough, click on **Home** button on the toolbar.

4.1.2.2 tips and tricks for better searching

All sites have a search box for you to type keyword(s), but each site works a bit differently. Hence, it's a good idea to learn to use the site you are searching. A little time spent on reading the help menu to determine how to search on keywords can save you hours of frustrations. To make your search more successful, here are ten tips and tricks you can use which most web directories or search engines will understand (and those that don't will generally ignore them).

10 tricks and tips for better searching

Note Be careful about using quote marks. Some sites will accept the words in quotes; others prefer the words to be linked by a Boolean Operator like AND, OR, NOT. For more information on Boolean Operators see Section 4.2.1.

Also do remember that while some search engines like AltaVista and others allow the use of symbols, most search engines will require you to use linking words like AND, OR, NOT.

1 **Have a plan** – Before starting a search, prepare a list of appropriate keywords, synonyms and phrases relating to the topic you are researching. Be specific. The more precise you can be, the better the results will be.

2 **Use multiple keywords** – If you want to search for something that can't be encapsulated in a single word then you can enter several keywords, but do type the most important keyword followed by the least important. For example, if you wanted to find 'research studies in nursing', type nursing research. This list will present good links to nursing sites before the rather more general links to sites, which only contain research studies.

3 **Use lower case letters** – Keywords entered in lower case characters are generally case insensitive, while those entered with capital letters make the search case sensitive. So, use upper case or block characters only if you expect to find upper case characters. For example, searching for 'DISEASE' may find very little, but searching for 'Disease' or 'disease' should find a lot.

4 **Use quote marks** – To find a particular phrase, try enclosing it in 'quote marks'. A search for 'Anorexia Nervosa' would find only pages containing this phrase and ignore pages that just contain one word or the other.

5 **Prefix your keyword with symbols** – You can broaden or narrow your search by prefixing your keyword with a '+' sign if it must be included, with a '−' sign if it must be excluded and 'l' sign if you want everything. For example, if you're searching for *Insomnia in men*, you type +insomnia men −women. Similarly, you type tumours −benign to ensure that you did not find pages about benign tumours. Or, you could type tumours malignant lbenign to ensure both types are included. (See Section 4.2.1.1)

6 **Avoid using plural words** – Most search engines tend to search on substrings. For example, if you use the keyword disease, they will return hits on diseases, but searching for diseases might miss relevant information on Paget's disease.

7 **Use wildcards** – If, for example, you are searching for information about nursing, you can search on 'nurs*' to cover *nurse, nurses, nursing*. Do remember that the symbols for wildcards vary depending on the search engine you are using. AltaVista uses an asterisk.

8 **Try synonyms** – If you are looking for information on pressure sore, search on *ulcer, wound, bedsore*. . . .

9 **Use alternative spellings** – Sometimes it is wise when carrying out a particular search to try multiple spellings. For example, try *disk, disc*. If you are researching schizophrenia, try *catatonia, catatonic, katanonia, katatonic*.

10 **Be persistent, creative and resourceful** – As the saying goes, if at first you don't succeed try again. Use different search tools and databases. How successful you are with your search depends on your knowledge and skill at using the technology.

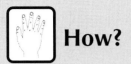

How?

how to set search options

Yahoo! UK & Ireland will normally search categories, titles and comments to find listings that contain all of your keywords. Equally, Yahoo! will not pay attention to case (e.g. 'National Meningitis Trusts' is treated just like 'national meningitis trusts') and will stop after it finds 100 matches. However, you can customize your search. You can specify:

- Whether you want matches to contain all of your keywords or at least one of your keywords;
- Whether your keywords should be considered as substrings or whole words;
- The number of matches displayed per page.

4.1.2.3 search results

Yahoo! searches retrieve the following three different kinds of information:

- Categories that match your keywords
- Web sites that match your keywords
- Categories where those sites are listed.

Thus, you can choose to go directly to retrieve sites, or browse around relevant categories for related information.

4.1.2.4 browsing yahoo!'s web directory

While carrying out the previous activity, you may have noticed that below the Yahoo! textbox into which you typed your keywords, there was a collection of hypertext links offering broad categories, which you can use to dig deeper to find more specific information (see Fig. 4.1).

Fig. 4.1 Hypertext links
A list of hypertext links offering broad categories, which can be used to dig deeper for more specific information

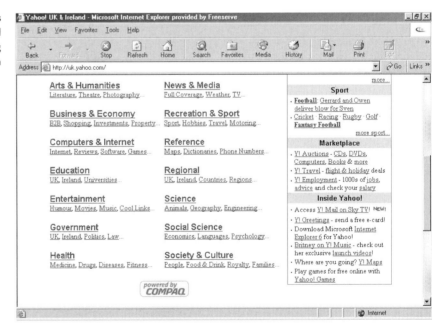

When you carry out the activity below, you would no doubt discover how easy it is to follow the Yahoo! layout. Yahoo! has used bold and plain text to help you navigate intelligently. Bold text means this is a link to another Yahoo! category; plain text indicates that it's a link to a page elsewhere on the web that contains the kind of information you have been searching for.

Activity 4.2 browsing yahoo! UK and Ireland

In the previous activity we had a particular Internet site in mind. We were looking for sites dealing with a medical condition called meningitis. Since we knew exactly what we wanted we were able to use the Search facility. But what if we did not have a particular Internet site in mind? In such a case we could have used the Browse facility to 'surf' the net and see what is there. To do this, we simply point and click on a topic we want to browse.

Before reading on, it is suggested that you carry out the steps listed in **Worksheet 6**.

When you have completed the activity return to this page and read on.

Worksheet 6 browsing with yahoo!'s web directory

1 If you are not logged on, re-start your browser and . . .
2 Enter the following URL in the Location/Address box:

   http://www.yahoo.co.uk

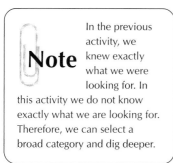

Note In the previous activity, we knew exactly what we were looking for. In this activity we do not know exactly what we are looking for. Therefore, we can select a broad category and dig deeper.

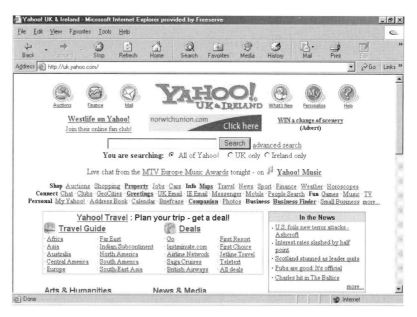

3 Point and click on the category 'Health'. (If you can't see it, use the scrollbar to move down.) *A new page should appear displaying a list of subcategories.*
4 Now, point and click on any sub-category of your choice. *This should move you to yet another page.*
5 If the page does not interest you, click on the **Back** button on your browser's toolbar to return to the sub-category list and try a different one. When you have had enough, click on **Home** button on the toolbar.

Take a look at the screen shot in Fig. 4.2. You should be able to see a number in brackets next to each of the categories. You may have already encountered this feature and wondered what it means. This number tells you how many links you can expect to find in that category. For example, in the category Diseases and Conditions I found 5573 links.

Fig. 4.2 Browsing
The screenshot on the right shows sub-headings with number of links in brackets

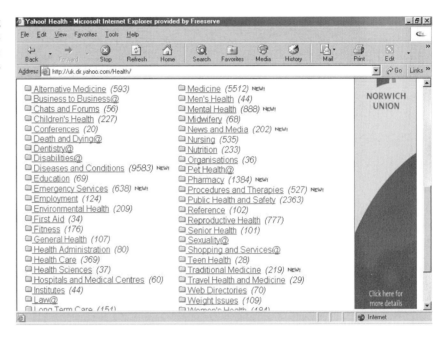

4.1.3 search engines

Search engines are the most sophisticated tools you can use to find information on the net. They use an automated piece of software (*Robot*) that visits web sites and follows their links. The search engines then index the full-text (or at least a significant part of the text) of all these pages in their database and allow users to search it by typing in keywords or subject terms. They may index millions of web pages but no single search engine indexes every web site on the Internet.

Furthermore, each search engine works a little differently and gathers a different collection of raw data. So when you send a search engine looking for a keyword, the results will vary depending on which search engine you use. While they are easy to use, you may have to learn to use several of them to find what you want. The search engines may also find links that look ideal, but turn out to be dead or unavailable when you go to use them. Pages go up and down on the web more quickly than the search engines can update their databases.

All search engines have huge databases, and quite often return long lists of matches or 'hits'. Sifting through them all can be quite daunting and time consuming. In a way, thousands of hits can be almost as useless as no hits at all. It is, therefore, imperative that you develop a few strategies and learn a few tricks to get more manageable results. In Section 4.1.2.2 above I have given you ten tips and tricks to help make your search a little easier. For more searching tips, pay a visit to:

http://www.wfi.fr/volterre/searchtips.html

You can access a search engine by typing its URL in the Address/Location box. The number of search engines is growing. Table 4.2 lists the most popular ones. The first three are specific to health-related information. Until recently the best search tools were available free of charge. Since some of them now require a subscription fee, some of the tools listed below may not be available for you to use on your college or organization computer network.

Table 4.2
Search engines

Note For a list of resources of articles and sites comparing Search engines, please visit

http://www.hamline.edu/library/bush/handouts/comparisons.html

Medical World Search	http://www.mwsearch.com/ This search engine was specially developed for the medical field. It indexes the full content of the major medical sites on the web, enabling users to search for any word in any of the pages indexed. It supports the use of Boolean operators: AND and OR. It allows for phrase and word group searching. Once a search is complete, a list of related and more specific words appear, at this point you can change your search using Boolean operators and terms from the thesaurus. For example, typing the keyword 'disease' produces 34147 documents, entering the keyword 'diseases in twins' (a thesaurus term) produces a more precise two documents. Before you can use this system you must register yourself as a user and pay a small fee of £10/year.
Mirago Health	http://health.mirago.co.uk This is a UK-biased medical search engine providing authoritative information and a full web search facility for medical sites.
MedHunt	http://www.hon.ch/MedHunt/ This is a specialist full-text search engine developed by Health on the Net (HON) that focuses on health/medical web sites. MedHunt also functions as a web directory.
Lycos	http://www.lycos.com This is one of the first and biggest search engines. It claims to have indexed 91 per cent of the Web. Although better search engines have since appeared, it remains comprehensive, dependable and easy to use, though it is somewhat slow. The index searches by document title, links and keywords. It offers many search options and returns a ranked list with options for terse or long display. It is often busy. It allows the use of wildcard. To expand a word with wildcard, you add the symbol $ symbol to the end of the word, e.g. *commun*$ to get *communicate*, and *communication*. You can use the period (.) after a word to prohibit its expansion: for example, ***washing.*** to avoid ***Washington.***
HotBot	http://www.hotbot.com This is a highly recommended search engine. It has over 54 million documents. It is up to date and incredibly fast. It offers a list of options to help you refine your searches, one of which allows you to use Boolean operators.
AltaVista	http://www.altavista.digital.com This search engine started in 1995 and has over 8 billion words covering over 30 million web pages. It is comprehensive and consistently returns useful information at lightning speed. It allows you to conduct simple or advanced searches and you can have

Table 4.2 (*cont.*)		the results listed in summary or detailed form. You can also use a wildcard when searching AltaVista. The wildcard symbol is the asterisk (*), and means 'anything can go here'. For example, if you are looking for information on schizophrenia, you could type in the search box Schizo* to ensure you get hits that include the words Schizo-affective disorder, schizoid personality disorder, schizoid innovations, etc. For tips on searching with AltaVista, visit http://www.topwebsite.co.uk/altavista.shtml
	Excite	http://www.excite.com This search engine has full text to over 11.5 million pages and is updated weekly. It is different from other search engines in that it searches not only by keyword, but by concept. It uses 'fuzzy logic'. In other words it tries to find *what* you want and not just what you say you want. Like AltaVista, Excite also lets you use the plus sign or minus sign in front of a word rather than use the Boolean operators AND, or AND NOT.
	Infoseek **and** **InfoSeek** **Ultra**	http://www.infoseek.com and http://ultra.infoseek.com InfoSeek is a valuable search tool. It allows for phrase searching, which greatly increases the quality of your results. It also has a guide to the 'best of the Web'. Infoseek also allows you to search FAQs (lists of Frequently asked Questions), which can be very useful places to start researching a topic. InfoSeek Ultra is fast and furious. InfoSeek UltraSmart is a cross between a search engine and a web directory. See Table 4.1
	Web **Crawler**	http://www.webcrawler.com This search engine is fast, relatively easy to use, indexes titles as well as content, recently absorbed by American Online, and returns a ranked list of hits with no descriptions. It includes a list of the 25 most visited sites on the web. It is not nearly as comprehensive as other search engines. It allows the use of AND, OR and NOT in the standard search field. For better results, items may also be grouped within parentheses: depression AND NOT (manic or adolescent)

4.1.3.1 carrying out a search using a search engine

Most search engines look much the same and although they work in slightly different ways, the basic principles are the same. For our next activity let's use Lycos. When you run Lycos, you'll see a page similar to the one shown in the screenshot below (Fig. 4.3).

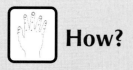

How?

How to select the right search engine to use

Deciding which one to choose is difficult, as there is no known single search tool that can satisfy every query. However, connection difficulties will often make this choice for you. As you start using these tools you will soon find out that Lycos is rarely available during working hours. WebCrawler is more often available, is easy to use, and as a consequence will often be your first choice. InfoSeek has been favourably reviewed and rated number one in several recent studies. Excite and the others are also worth exploring. Here are a few points to bear in mind:

- When using a search engine you must know what you are looking for, as you have to create your own search terms.
- Information gathered by search engines is done automatically with no human intervention. Hence there is no quality control.
- When you are using a search engine you are only searching the pages indexed and found by the search engine you are using.
- Different search engines work in slightly different ways and offer different search options. The available search options are usually detailed in Help pages associated with each search engine. So do make an effort to read these. Knowing how best to organize your search terms can save time and greatly improve your search results.
- Different search engines are better for some searches than others. For example, WebCrawler is an inappropriate tool for an author or name search, but its full page indexing can be very effective when looking for an obscure term.
- WebCrawler indexes every word of a web page, while the Lycos index is built with only selected words, such as the title, the headings, and the most significant 100 words. These differences contribute to the very different result sets that are returned by different search engines for the same query.
- Make a point of using one or two search engines regularly so that you can become familiar with each one's specific searching techniques.

Fig. 4.3 The Lycos homepage
This is the starting page for Lycos. To search the web, simply type your keyword or keywords in the textbox and then press the **Enter** key on your keyboard.
After you have typed a keyword (or keywords) into the textbox, press the **Enter** key on your keyboard. Your browser will send the information off to the engine

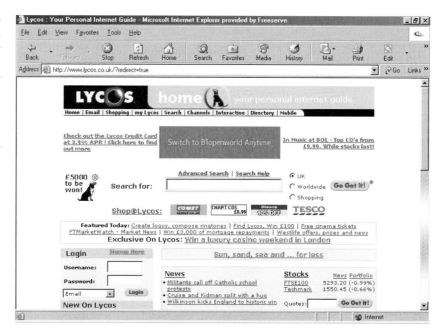

Activity 4.3 exploring a web site using lycos

To compare Lycos with Yahoo!, let's once again attempt to find information on the medical condition meningitis.

For hands-on experience, follow the steps listed in **Worksheet 7**.

When you have completed the activity return to this page and read on.

Worksheet 7 searching with lycos

When you arrive at the Lycos site you will see a page like the one shown in the screenshot. You will notice it is not so dissimilar to Yahoo!. It has a search engine textbox into which you can type keywords. Since we know exactly what we are looking for (i.e. information on meningitis), we can use this textbox to do a search.

1 Log on to Windows and start your browser.
2 Enter the following URL in the Location/Address box:

http://www.lycos.com

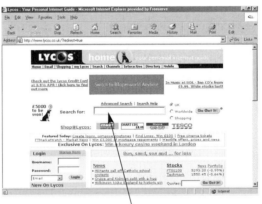

3 Point and click in this textbook. *A flashing cursor should appear.*
4 Type the keyword: **meningitis**, then click the **Find** button. *After a few seconds you should see a new page listing the first ten sites that matched your search criteria. (You may need to scroll down ↓ to see the list.)*

Fig. 4.4 Search criteria

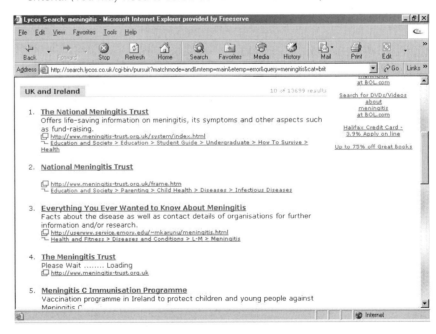

5 Click on any of the links that interest you. If the page does not interest you, click on the **Back** button on your browser's toolbar to return to the search results and try a different one. When you have had enough, click on the **Home** button on the toolbar.

Note An ill-defined search could result in 100s of sites being identified – most of which may not be relevant. For example, as shown in the screenshot opposite, a search on the keyword 'meningitis' found 13699 related web pages. If you find that too many sites have been identified, it is most likely that you have not defined your search criteria well enough. You should try again using more specific keywords or keyphrases.

Once you have looked at the first ten you can go to the next ten, then the next and so on. If you have followed a link and you are not satisfied with the content you can go back. Just click on the **Back** button on the browser's toolbar.

Some search engines give the pages a score for relevancy. As a rule of thumb you should only consider pages with a score of 75% or above. If you can't find what you are looking for with one search engine, always try another. Different search engines use different methods of searching and can produce different results. To experience the differences do the next activity.

Activity 4.4 exploring a web site using alternative search engines

Now carry out a few searches using the other search engines listed in Table 4.2 above.

When you have completed the activity return to this page and read on.

If after completing this section you still feel you need more help on using search engines, pay a visit to this web site:

http://daphne.palomar.edu/TGSEArch

4.1.4 information gateways for health and medical sources

Gateway: a program or device that acts as a kind of translator between two networks that wouldn't otherwise be able to communicate with each other. Subject gateways provide access to evaluated web sites that can support learning and research, but the site coverage is relatively small.

Anyone can publish on the net. It is, therefore, not surprising that the Internet is packed with all sorts of information. The down side is that as there is no quality control, most of the available information has not been evaluated. To deal with the problems of quality and quantity, Information **Gateways** have been developed. Gateways facilitate Internet browsing and searching and are specifically designed to help you find high-quality Internet sites and resources. Some of these gateways have been funded by Higher Education in the United Kingdom.

Information Gateways are different from search engines, as they are more like an online catalogue for the Internet; i.e. they will only have details of the very best web links in a particular subject. The process of filtering is carried out by a team of experts employed for that purpose. This enables them to offer unrivalled quality control, with each Internet site being hand-picked, described and classified. They are often geared to support academic learning and research communities. Some gateways specialise in particular subjects while others cover a range of subjects.

Exploring the Internet is rather like diving into an electronic boot fair: the information gateways can be a very useful starting point. As a student of health care you should find the five information gateways listed in Table 4.3 quite useful.

Table 4.3	**NHS**	This is the only membership body for all NHS organizations. To access this gateway you enter this URL in the Location/ Address box in your browser: http://www.nhsconfed.net (See Subsection 4.1.4.1.)
Information (or subject) gateways	**Confederation**	
	OMNI	http://omni.ac.uk (Acronym for Organizing Medical Networked Information). This is a UK-based subject gateway to high-quality Internet resources in medicine, biomedicine, allied health, health management, and related topics. All sites found through this gateway have been evaluated and indexed and come with a brief description that enables you to assess their usefulness before you visit. (See Subsection 4.1.4.2.)
	SOSIG (pronounced sausage)	http://www.sosig.ac.uk (Short for Social science Information Gateway.) It contains approximately 5000 high-quality information resources for social scientists to use. (See Subsection 4.1.4.3.)
	HON	http://www.hon.ch/ (Short for Health On the Net.) Quite similar to OMNI. Contents of each site have been reviewed and supplemented by an automatically generated database. (See Subsection 41.4.4.)
	NMAP	http://nmap.ac.uk (Short for Nursing, Midwifery and Allied Professionals.) It is the UK's gateway to high-quality Internet resources in Nursing, Midwifery and Allied Health. (See Subsection 4.1.4.5.)
	Medical Matrix	http://www.medmatrix.org/ This is a free online directory of selected medical sites on the Internet, with a primary audience of health care professionals. It provides annotated pointers to a comprehensive database of global resources that can assist in patient care. It specializes in clinical resources and provides a useful starting point for some initial Internet exploration. This directory is more aimed at US doctors and health care workers, and requires registration. (See Subsection 4.1.4.6.)

4.1.4.1 nhs confederation

To access the NHS Confederation you simply enter this URL in the Location/ Address box of your browser:

http://www.nhsconfed.net/

When you reach the NHS gateway homepage you have to choose England, Wales, Scotland or Northern Ireland. This will take you to the main page from where you can select various resources. You can sign on to the NHS Confederation Extranet, or you can click on **Useful Links**. The latter will take you to a wide selection of useful links on the web. Table 4.4 shows the possibilities:

Fig. 4.5 The NHS gateway

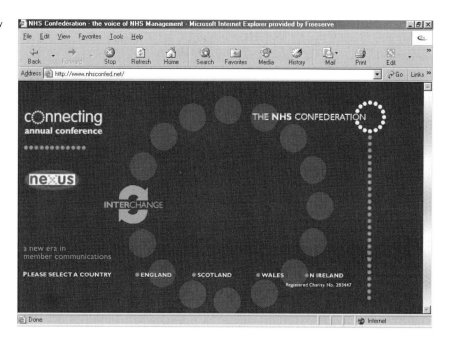

Table 4.4

Useful links on the web

Subject area	Contains links to the following web sites
The NHS on the Internet	NHS Direct online The Department of Health, Social Services and Public Safety
Health organizations on the web	Department of Health Chief Executives Bulletin (weekly) COIN: Circulars on the Internet Health and personal social services statistics in England (annual) Index to recent DoH publications National Plan NHS Performance Tables Statistics and Surveys (DoH)
Sites dedicated to clinical excellence	National Institute for Clinical Excellence A ScHARR Introduction to free databases of interest to NHS staff on the Internet Critical Appraisal Skills Programme (CASP)
Royal College, unions and associations	BMA RCN Unison TUC Health Financial Management Association
Health information sources	Electronic library for Social Care Electronic Medicines Compendium Learning Zone National Electronic Library for Health National Research Register

Table 4.4 (*cont.*)	Subject area	Contains links to the following web sites
	Health news sites	Bandolier
		BMJ
		Evening Standard
		Health Service Journal
		Nursing Standard
		The Lancet
		Newspapers: *The Times, Daily Telegraph, Financial Times*, etc.

4.1.4.2 omni

RDN is short for 'Resource Discovery Network' – an Internet search service designed for academics and professionals. It is the UK's centre for its national subject gateways, built with funding from the government and national research councils.

OMNI (Organizing Medical Networked Information) is another gateway to high-quality Internet resources in medicine, biomedicine, allied health, health management, and related topics. It is part of the BIOME hub, which belongs to the network of hubs established by the **RDN**. It provides comprehensive coverage of the UK resources in this area and access to the best resources worldwide. Using a process of selection, evaluation and description the collection is regularly updated. The OMNI databases were last updated 19 October 2001.

To use OMNI simply enter this URL in the Location/Address box of your browser:

http://omni.ac.uk

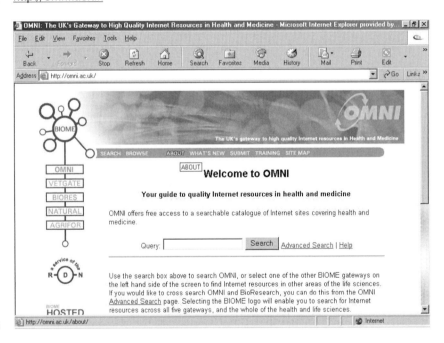

Fig. 4.6 The OMNI homepage

4.1.4.3 sosig

SOSIG (short for Social Science Information Gateway, was the first subject-based information gateway in the UK and was established in 1994. It is a free Internet service and contains approximately 500 high-quality Internet information for students, academics, researchers, and practitioners in the social sciences, business and law to use. The Internet resources cover a range of different formats from books, reports, newsletters, bibliographies, databases, mailing lists, and software. Table 4.5 below lists the range of subjects covered by SOSIG.

The SOSIG Internet Catalogue is structured in a way that allows you either to browse resource descriptions within subject headings or to use keyword searching of the descriptions. The SOSIG button bar is available at the top of every page and will help you navigate through the Gateway. To use SOSIG visit this URL:

http://www.sosig.ac.uk

Table 4.5
The range of subjects covered by SOSIG

Business (Accountancy, management . . .)	**Philosophy** (Ethics, Logic, Metaphysics . . .)
Economics (Finance, Trade and Commerce . . .)	**Politics** (International Relations, Political Parties . . .)
Education (Higher Education, Teaching Methods . . .)	**Psychology** (General, Social . . .)
Environmental Sciences and Issues (Protection of the Environment . . .)	**Social Science General** (Social Policy, Social Science Methodology . . .)
Ethnology, Ethnography, Anthropology (Teaching and Research . . .)	**Social Welfare** (adoption/Foster Care, Social Work . . .)
Geography (Economic, Social . . .)	**Sociology** (Schools and Theories, Sociologists . . .)
Government and Public Administration (Local Government, Policing . . .)	**Statistics** (Demography, Official Statistics . . .)
Law (By area, UK law . . .)	**Women's Studies** (Women and Employment, Women's History . . .)

4.1.4.4 health on the net (hon)

Fig. 4.7 The health on the net homepage

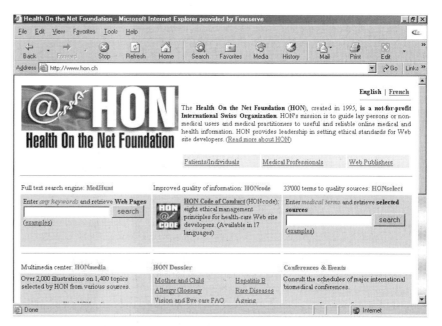

This is very similar to OMNI. The database has been created manually. The content of each site has been reviewed and supplemented by an automatically generated database. But, unlike OMNI, searching is automatically carried out across both databases. Search results are place into two categories: reviewed and unreviewed. It permits simple and advanced searching (Boolean operators, wildcards, phrase searching). In addition you will find a searchable database of medical images and movies, selected abstracts and full text papers from conferences and journals and information about conferences and events. To use this HON, type this URL in the Location/Address box of your browser:

http://www.hon.ch/

4.1.4.5   nmap

BIOME offers free access to a searchable catalogue of Internet sites and resources covering the health and life sciences. You can choose to search BIOME using the search box provided for Internet resources in the whole of the health and life sciences, or choose one of the five subject-specific gateways from the menu bar to the left of the screen. Unlike generic search engines, BIOME only directs you to Internet resources that have been hand selected and quality-evaluated. BIOME is funded by the Joint Information Systems Committee (JISC), and their target audience is the UK learning, teaching and research community. However, searching is free, and they hope they are also of value to users beyond their target community.

Do not confuse this with BIOMED

NMAP (Nursing, Midwifery and Allied Health Professions) is yet another gateway to evaluated, quality Internet resources. It is aimed at students, researchers, academics, and practitioners in the health and medical sciences. This gateway is the creation of a core team of information specialists and subject experts coordinated at the University of Nottingham Greenfield Medical Library, in partnership with key organizations throughout the UK. It was launched in April 2001. Content providers from relevant professional organizations help to ensure that NMAP meets the needs of the professions. It is closely integrated with the OMNI gateway.

NMAP is one of the gateways within the **BIOME** service (http://biome.ac.uk/). By the way, BIOME is funded by the Joint Information Systems Committee (JISC) (http://www.jics.ac.uk) through the Resource Discovery Network (RDN) (http://www.rdn.ac.uk).

In line with the philosophy of subject gateways, Internet resources available via NMAP have been selected for their quality and relevance to the nursing, midwifery and allied health professions. These resources have been reviewed and their descriptions are, in general, stored in a structured database. NMAP is yet another useful tool for accessing health resources on the net.

You can access NMAP by entering the following URL in the Location/Address box of your browser:

http://NMAP.ac.uk

4.1.4.6   medical matrix

This is another health and medical Information Gateway. It is a collection of selected medical sites that have been evaluated by a panel of physicians and medical librarians. Although this gateway does have a US bias, it nevertheless offers health professionals a good collection of evaluated resources. Before you can use this gateway you are required to complete an online registration form. You can use this gateway to:

• Browse Internet resources by topic
• Carry out clinical searches on key medical online databases
• Find resources which have been selected, ranked and peer-reviewed by health professionals
• Search for medical Internet resources using keywords.

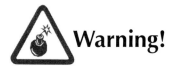**Warning!**

4 key points to remember when using Information Gateways

1 It is wise to use broader search terms than those you would use on a search engine, because the collections are smaller due to the amount of human effort required.
2 You are searching catalogue records which describe Internet resources that then direct you to relevant resources on the World Wide Web.
3 When you browse a Subject Gateway, although you are browsing a relatively small collection of resources, it is a high-quality collection.
4 Resource descriptions provided for each web site have usually been written by professionals or subject specialists. Read them and you will get a good idea of whether the site in question is suitable for your needs or not.

Activity 4.5 bookmarking sites of interest

- Visit the NHS Gateway. At the homepage select from the list offered a heading that interests you.
- Add NHS Gateway to your bookmark list. (For Help refer to Section 3.2.3 and Worksheet 4.)
- Visit the SOSIG Gateway and browse the resource descriptions within the subject headings.
- Add SOSIG Gateway to your bookmark list.
- Visit the HON gateway and browse the resource descriptions within the subject headings.
- Add HON Gateway to your hotlist.

Database searching using OMNI and NMAP

- Carry out the task set in **Worksheet 8**. You will find step-by-step instructions on how to carry out a basic search on OMNI.
- Using the URL given in Table 4.3 access NMAP. Then using the Browse facility, browse the RCN headings.

When you have completed the activity return to the next page and read on.

1 Log on to Windows and start your browser.
2 Enter the following URL in the Location/Address box:

http://omni.ac.uk

Fig. 4.8

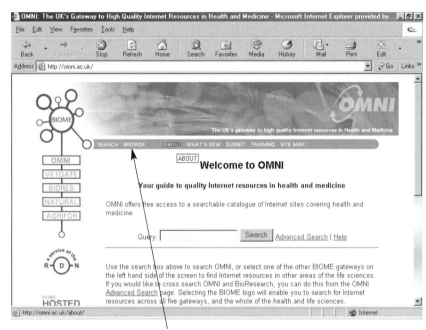

3 Click on the command **Browse**. *A list of categories should appear.*
4 Click on the command **Browse by NLM subject headings**. *Subject listings using NLM for OMNI should appear.*
5 Find the heading **Nursing** and click on it.
6 Scroll down and find **Evidence-based nursing**. Read what the description says and then click that link. *The homepage of this web site should appear.*
7 Click on the URL in the Address/Location box. *This should highlight the URL.*
8 Now, add to your hotlist/favourites.

This section has introduced you to three types of search tools that you can use to navigate the Information Superhighway, in the same way you might use a road map. It won't feature all the byways and side roads of the Internet, but will serve you as a basic navigational guide. Table 4.6 below provides a fair comparison of the tools.

Table 4.6
A comparison of the three discovery tools

Web Directories	Information Gateways	Search Engines
An example of a health Web Directory: Achoo (For more refer to Table 4.1)	An example of a health Information Gateway: NMAP (For more refer to Table 4.3)	An example of a health Search Engine: MedHunt (For more refer to Table 4.2)
Use human editors to organize their Internet resources but quality control can vary from a lot to none.	Use a combination of an automated program and human editors (subject specialists) to filter and organize their Internet resources.	An index of web pages is created automatically by a special program. Nobody checks whether the information on any site is correct or whether it is useful. Hence no quality control.
Most directories are aimed at the general public; therefore they will include popular, recreational and commercial sites.	Provides a description of the resource available on each web site. The descriptions are usually written by information professionals or subject specialists.	Most search engines cater for the general market and will include recreational, popular commercial and educational resources.
When searching a web directory, you should use broader terms than you would use on a search engine, because the collection is small.	When searching an information gateway, you should use broader terms, because the collection is small. Remember you are not searching the actual resources themselves. You are searching catalogue records that describe Internet resources.	To use a search engine you must know what you are looking for as you have to create your own search terms. With most search engines you can use Boolean operators to combine key words or key phrases.
When browsing a web directory, remember that large subject hierarchies may take a lot of browsing and the headings may not be as useful as you would like.	When browsing an information gateway, remember although the collection is small it is of a high quality.	No single search engine indexes every web site on the Internet. You are only searching the pages indexed and found by the search engine you are using. Search engines give you the biggest number of results, but a lot of what they find might not be of any use. Some offer a browsable listing of resources.
Useful to browse through the Internet when you are not sure what you are looking for.	These are the best tools to use when you want to start exploring what's available on the Internet.	Use a search engine when you know what you are looking for.
Also useful when you are looking for specific organization, as they are easily categorized and can usually be found quite quickly using a hierarchical browsing structure.	Provides access to evaluated web sites that can support learning and research, but the site coverage is relatively small.	You need to be able to evaluate the worth of the material found by search engines.

The range of *databases* available to health students and staff has grown at an alarming rate. To provide a detailed explanation of each is beyond the scope of this unit. Some of the possibilities are CINAHL (Cumulative Index of Nursing and Allied Health Literature) and Medline. Both of these databases are important resources to help you keep up to date with new developments in health literature.

CINAHL and Medline are usually described as bibliographic databases because the records on these databases are mostly just references to published material. The most common publication types are articles published in professional/academic journals. However, the trend is for some databases to include access to full-text material, as distinct from just the reference.

Here are two examples of what a record on a bibliographic database might look like. The first example is a record of a published book, the second example is a record of a published journal article.

Example 1	**A record of a published book**
Accessions number	007
Author's name	Chellen, S.S.
Book title	Information Technology for the Caring Professions: a user's handbook
Publisher	Cassell
Publication year	1995
Publication type	Book
Subject heading 1	Computers, Nursing
Subject heading 2	History of Computing
Subject heading 3	Information Technology

Example 2	**A record of a published journal article**
Accessions number	008
Author's name	Chellen, S.S.
Article title	A Layman's Guide to IT
Publisher	Occupational Health: a Journal for Occupational Health Nurses 47 (10), 351–2, 354–5
Publication year	1995
Publication type	Journal article
Subject heading 1	Occupational Health
Subject heading 2	Information Technology
Subject heading 3	Databases
Subject heading 4	Computers

Each line indicated in the above records represents a different sort of information, i.e. *accession number*, *author's name*, *title*, *publisher*, *date of publication*, *type of publication*, and *subject headings*. Each line (aspect) is called a field. So you can see from the previous tables that both publications have the year 1995 in the field labelled 'Publication Year'.

Imagine you were doing a search on a database that contains the two records shown above. If you type in the Search box the keyword **Information Technology**, both records will be found because both have a field with the words Information Technology recorded. However, if you were to type the keyword **Databases**, only the journal article would be found as there is no specific mention of databases in the record for the book by Sydney S. Chellen.

On CINAHL and Medline subject headings, which are added to the records, enhance the reference by describing accurately what it is about. The choice of subject headings will vary from database to database. For example, one health database may use the term Old Age, another may use the term Aged. Therefore to do a search for Elderly is not likely to be as successful, in terms of records found. How do you know then?

Some database services will map your term to the best subject headings on the database relevant. This allows some assistance to you when searching, as it will help to format the search strategy. Otherwise it is a good idea to be thinking laterally about your search, i.e. think of alternative words or expressions to use when searching a subject.

With the development of compact discs the trend in the information world was to store databases on compact discs called CD-ROMs. Since the escalation of the use of the Internet, a range of commercial databases, increasingly with full-text services, is becoming available through this channel. One of the leading electronic information retrieval services is Ovid Technologies Inc. CINAHL and Medline are just two examples of databases that were only available on CD-ROM, but now have become available on the Net. (For more information see Unit 1, under the heading: Databases.)

There are advantages and limitations with every database so it is practical to become competent with a number of different search tools when researching a subject. There are still benefits in adopting the traditional hand searching of the journals literature. This is especially important with the latest copies of a journal title. Remember it can be several months before a reference published in a journal will be available on a bibliographic database and even then not everything which is published in any particular journal issue would end up on a database.

Activity 4.6 what's available

Although more and more electronic databases are becoming available for use, do not expect to be able to have access to all of them at your local health, college/university or professional library/computing laboratory. Use this checklist to tick (✓) those that are available at your institution and establish if they are on CD-ROMs or part of the Ovid–Biomed service.

☐ Medline
☐ CINAHL
☐ Cancerlit
☐ Core Biomedical Collection
☐ EBM reviews – ACP Journal Club
☐ Mental Health Collection
☐ Nursing Collection
☐ Cochrane Database of Systematic reviews
☐ Cochrane Controlled Trials register
☐ Database of Abstracts of Reviews of Effectiveness
☐ British Nursing Index (BNI)
☐ PsycINFO.

When you have completed the activity return to the next page and read on.

Most databases allow for the facility to combine terms together using special linking words often called Boolean Operators. These special words (or Boolean Operators) are: AND, OR and NOT. The best way to think of these is to imagine they are like doing equations with words.

Each operator is explained below and is visually described using Venn diagrams.

QUERY 1, using the operator **AND**

Let's say you are interested in the relationship between '**nursing**' and '**stress**' and would like to find relevant information. You can combine both keywords with the operator AND, e.g. nursing AND stress. By doing so, you will narrow your search and retrieve only records/documents in which BOTH search terms are present. This is illustrated by the **shaded** area overlapping the two circles in the Venn diagram below representing all the records that contain both the keyword 'nursing' and the keyword 'stress'. Notice how we do not retrieve any records/documents with only 'nursing' or only 'stress'.

Fig. 4.9

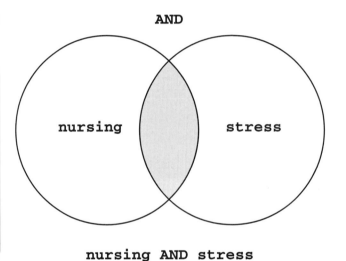

AND

nursing   stress

nursing AND stress

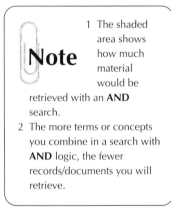

Note

1 The shaded area shows how much material would be retrieved with an **AND** search.
2 The more terms or concepts you combine in a search with **AND** logic, the fewer records/documents you will retrieve.

Here is an example of how AND logic works:

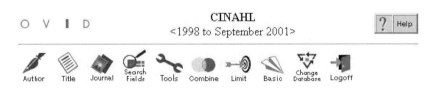

OVID   CINAHL   ? Help
              <1998 to September 2001>

Author Title Journal Search Tools Combine Limit Basic Change Logoff
                        Fields   Database

#	Search History	Results	Display
1	nursing.mp.	22929	Display
2	STRESS/ or stress.mp.	3562	Display
3	(nursing and stress).mp. [mp=title, cinahl subject heading, abstract, instrumentation]	387	Display

Suppose you would like information on '**nursing**' or '**midwifery**'. You can combine both keywords with the operator OR, e.g. nursing OR midwifery. By doing so, you will broaden your search and retrieve records/documents in which AT LEAST ONE of the search terms is present. This is illustrated in the Venn diagram below by:

- The **shaded** circle with the word **nursing** representing all the records/ documents that contain the keyword 'nursing'
- The shaded circle with the word **midwifery** representing all the records/ documents that contain the keyword 'midwifery'
- The shaded overlap area representing all the records/documents that contain both 'nursing' and 'midwifery'.

> **Note**
>
> 1 The shaded area shows how much material would be retrieved with an **OR** search.
> 2 **OR** logic is most commonly used to search for synonymous terms or concepts.
> 3 **OR** logic collates the results to retrieve all the unique records/documents of one term, the other, or both.
> 4 The more terms or concepts you combine in a search with **OR** logic, the more records/documents you will retrieve.

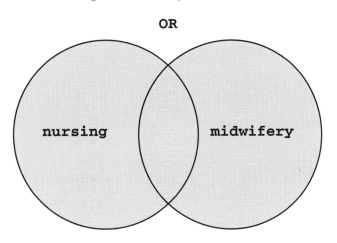

OR

nursing OR midwifery

Fig. 4.10

Here is an example of how OR logic works:

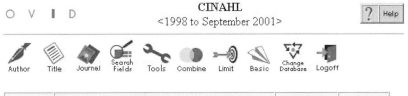

#	Search History	Results	Display
1	nursing.mp.	22929	Display
2	midwifery.mp. or MIDWIFERY/	2440	Display
3	(nursing or midwifery).mp. [mp=title, cinahl subject heading, abstract, instrumentation]	25069	Display

QUERY 3, using the operator **NOT**

OK, you would like to find information on '**nursing**', but want to avoid retrieving anything about '**midwifery**'. You can combine both keywords with the operator NOT, e.g. nursing NOT midwifery. By doing so, you will eliminate from your search all records/documents containing the keyword 'midwifery' and retrieve records/documents which contain the keyword 'nursing'. This is illustrated in the Venn diagram below by:

- The shaded area with the word **nursing** representing all the records/documents containing the keyword 'nursing'.
- No records/documents are retrieved in which the word 'midwifery' appears, even if the word 'nursing' appears there too.

Fig. 4.11

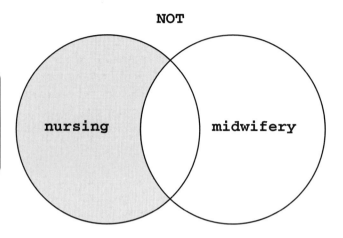

NOT

`nursing NOT midwifery`

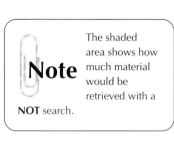

Note The shaded area shows how much material would be retrieved with a **NOT** search.

Here is an example of how **NOT** logic works:

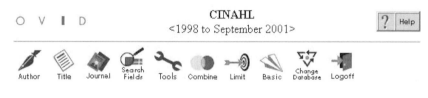

O V I D   CINAHL
<1998 to September 2001>

#	Search History	Results	Display
1	nursing.mp.	22929	Display
2	midwifery.mp. or MIDWIFERY/	2440	Display
3	(nursing not midwifery).mp. [mp=title, cinahl subject heading, abstract, instrumentation]	22629	Display

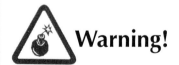

Warning! **NOT** logic excludes records/documents from your search results. Be careful when you use NOT: the term you do want may be present in an important way in documents that also contain the word you wish to avoid.

4.2.1.1 boolean searching on the internet

The Internet is a vast computer database. As such, its contents can be searched using the principles of Boolean logic. Many search engines offer the option to do full Boolean searching, i.e. allowing the use of the Boolean logical operators like AND, OR and NOT. Some search engines, such as Excite, defaults to OR. But many well-known search engines that traditionally defaulted to OR logic are moving away from that practice.

Another area of Boolean logic that is becoming a more common standard is 'implied Boolean logic'. In implied Boolean logic, symbols are used to represent Boolean logical operators. Table 4.7 below shows three examples of implied Boolean logic.

Table 4.7
Implied Boolean logic

Query 1: You want information about **pressure sores**:
    Boolean logic: OR
    Keyword Search   sores ulcers
    In the above example, some search engines will interpret the space between the two keywords as the Boolean operator OR.

Query 2: You are interested in obtaining information about **anorexia in men**:
    Boolean logic: AND
    Keyword Search   +anorexia +men

Query 3: You want information about **radiation, but not nuclear radiation**:
    Boolean logic: NOT
    Keyword Search   Radiation −nuclear

4.2.1.2 searching by keyphrase

You do not always have to use *keywords*. You can use *keyphrase*. Keyphrase enables you to search for words that appear together to make a phrase. When using a keyphrase you should enclose all the words in quotes, e.g. 'pressure sores'. In this example only literature containing this phrase will be found. Those that contain the word 'pressure' or 'sores' will be ignored.

4.2.1.3 searching using truncation or wildcards

Another searching technique is to use truncation. For example if you are searching for information about nursing, you can search on nurs* to cover *nurse, nurses, nursing*. Truncation will find variations of words such as plurals and similar words with different endings. You should use truncation with care as it will find much more material in areas that may not be pertinent. (Do remember that symbols for wildcards vary depending on the search engine you are using. AltaVista uses an asterisk.)

4.2.2 planning and undertaking an electronic search

Do not make the mistake of rushing online and start typing words or phrases in search boxes. This is usually quite unproductive. A successful online literature search requires planning. The more care and thought you put in planning how you will look for information, the more relevant your search results will be. A well-designed plan will:

• Save you time in the long run
• Enable you to search for information in many different places
• Help you to find a larger amount of *relevant* information.

A useful technique is to utilize a problem-solving approach, as this offers a systematic and organized method of electronic literature searching. Take a look at the following steps:

Fig. 4.12 Steps in undertaking an electronic search

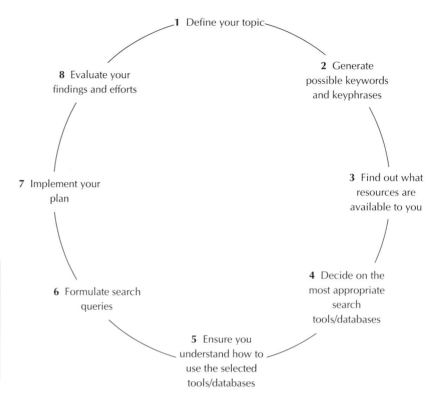

1 Define your topic

2 Generate possible keywords and keyphrases

3 Find out what resources are available to you

4 Decide on the most appropriate search tools/databases

5 Ensure you understand how to use the selected tools/databases

6 Formulate search queries

7 Implement your plan

8 Evaluate your findings and efforts

Note The best time to search the net in the UK is when America is asleep. So, try searching in the early morning and evening. This way you will avoid heavy Internet traffic.

Let's imagine you would like to find information on '**Pressure sores**'. This is how this might work.

1 Define your topic

- In this first step you must be very clear what it is that you are looking for, i.e. what information you need to answer your query and write them down. For example, if you've chosen a topic like 'pressure sores', as it stands it is too broad. To find *relevant* information, you need to refine your query. You can do this by asking yourself a few questions.

Fig. 4.13 An illustration of how a topic can be translated into a workable query statement

1 Are you looking for general information on pressure sores or are you, for instance, more interested in research articles? If it is the latter, then a more useful query statement would be:

Research articles on pressure sores

2 Are you looking for research articles that relate to the care of a specific group, e.g. elderly male patients. Then your query statement would be:

Research articles on care of pressure sores in elderly male patients

3 Are you looking for research materials in specific journals, e.g. UK journals? Then your query statement would look like this:

Research materials published in UK journals on the care of pressure sores in elderly male patients

4 Are you interested in a specific aspect of care of pressure sores, e.g. the use of the Norton scale in assessing pressure sores? Then your query statement would be:

Research materials published in UK journals on the use of the Norton scale in assessing pressure sores in elderly male patients

5 Are you looking for bibliographical references to materials or do you want full text or both?

(Note: Databases like CINAHL, MEDLINE, CANCERLIT are bibliographical databases. Using these databases, all you should expect is a list of references and an abstract. To obtain the actual article, you will need to go to the source or a full-text database.)

- So the focus of your query is:

Research materials published in UK journals on the use of the Norton scale in assessing pressure sores in elderly male patients.

2 Generate possible keywords and keyphrases

Now that you're clear what you are looking for, you need to break down your query statement into its key parts and concepts. This will help you think of all possible keywords or keyphrases that are likely to help you with your search, particularly when searching in databases. Although at this stage different people may come up with different keywords/keyphrases and will finish off with slightly different search strategies and outcomes, what matters here is that you get the information you want.

For example to find information on:

Research materials published in UK journals on the use of **Norton scale** in assessing **pressure sores** in **elderly** male patients.

you should include in your search statement the concepts written in **bold** and you should use available features in the database/search tool to focus your search on those concepts that are underlined.

To increase the likelihood of finding relevant material, you also need to identify alternative keywords/phrases that describe the same concepts. You should think of:

- Synonyms (e.g. nurture, tending, attention)
- Plural/singular forms (e.g. man, men)
- Spelling variations (e.g. catatonic, katatonic)
- Acronyms (e.g. National Health Service, NHS).

Remember that many webpages and databases (like CINAHL) are produced in the US and therefore favour North American spelling and terminology.

Here are some alternatives for the concepts in the query statement: 'Research materials published in UK journals on the use of the **Norton scale** in assessing **pressure sores** in **elderly** male patients'.

Table 4.8

Concepts	Alternatives
Norton scale	Clinical assessment tools
	Risk assessment
	Risk factor
	Instrument validation
Pressure sores	Decubitus ulcer
	Bed sores
	Pressure ulcers
	Skin ulcers
Elderly	Old
	Aged
	mature

Tip: A useful way to find a list of keywords/keyphrases and alternative terms is to brainstorm with your friends.

3 Find out what resources are available to you

Once you are clear what you are searching for, you need to decide where to search. Not every all resources on the net are free and do not expect to have access to all available electronic journals and databases at your institution. So,

- Establish what fee-paying Internet services in your subject area your institution subscribes to
- Find out if you need to register yourself and obtain a username and password in order to use the services.

Tip: Ask the computing services or your librarian if you will be able to bookmark web sites when using PCs in the computing lab.

Many sites require online registration even if they are free. So, do keep a note of which passwords/usernames you need for each service you have registered for. If you lose or forget your password/username you will not be able to use the service until you have re-registered. Re-registration can take longer than you can afford to wait.

4 Decide on the most appropriate search tools/databases

Having ascertained that the Internet is the best place to look for the type of information you are after, you need to choose the right search tool(s)/database(s) for the job.

- Decide if you will be better off with a *search engine*, a *web directory* or an *information gateway*. (See Table 4.6.)
- Will an appropriate bibliographical database serve your needs or will you be better off searching a full-text database?
- Remember that search engines are good when you're looking for specific pieces of information, such as names and phrases. If you have broad or less-defined search terms, then web directories or Information Gateways are better as they will provide more accurate results and the information source have usually been vetted and described. (Read Subsections 4.1.2, 4.1.3 and 4.1.4.)

5 Ensure you understand how to use the selected tools/databases

To get the best out of search tools or databases you need to know how to use them. You need to know their idiosyncratic preferences:

- Which Boolean operators (AND, OR, NOT), if any, will you be able to use?
- Does the tool/database allow the use of implied Boolean logic, key-phrases , quotation marks (' '), or wildcards (* or $)? (Read Subsections 4.2.11, 4.2.1.2 and 4.2.1.3.)
- Read the help pages (that usually accompany search tools) to check for specific techniques on offer that might help to improve your search.

6 Formulate search queries

Spend some time thinking how you are going to use your list of keywords and keyphrases.

- Decide how you can group the keywords using Boolean operators AND, OR or NOT, or quotation marks. For example:
  'pressure sores'
  'Pressure sores' AND 'Norton scale'

- If you have decided to search a bibliographical database like CINAHL, do remember that it is an American bibliographical database. Thus, consider alternative terms such as, Bed sores, Pressure Ulcers, Skin ulcers, etc. For example:

  'Pressure sores' OR 'Bed sores' NOT 'Pressure Areas'

7 Implement your plan

Now it is time to put the plan into action.

- Locate/access your chosen tools/databases.
- Key in a search statement you have formulated.
- Use the features offered by the relevant database/search tool to focus your search, e.g. limit to <u>research articles</u>, <u>UK journals</u>, <u>male</u>.

Tip: Always start off with separate keywords then combine them later.

8 Evaluate your findings and efforts

You must determine how well the plan has worked and whether you need to make any changes in the plan or to refine your search strategies and skills. Try answering the following questions:

- Did you succeed in getting the information you wanted? If your initial searches did not find enough or too much information,not, are there additional search terms or keywords you could have tried to broaden or narrow your search? Are there alternative search tools and databases that you could try?
- Did you feel at ease using the chosen search tool(s) or database(s)?
- If you have used several search tools or databases, did you notice any differences?
- Did you have difficulties accessing the site or database?

Tip: As you come across sites you're interested in, if you can bookmark them, do so. (Read Subsection 3.2.3.) This will save time later on when you try to find them again by avoiding the trouble of having to write out the URL, which can be quite long. If this is not possible, make sure you note down the full URL of any Internet resources you find. Remember to copy them exactly, with attention to any punctuation and upper and lower case letters. A better way of ensuring accuracy is to copy and paste any URL into a word document.

If the Internet link did not work at the first attempt, check that you have entered the details correctly. Another tip is to enter just the root of the address. (Read 'Warning box' in Subsection 3.1.6.)

Note

Remember that you can print your finds or e-mail them to your box for later viewing.

Activity 4.7 writing a search statement

You have been given a task to research the truth about waiting lists in NHS Hospitals.

- Identify what are the keywords or keyphrases you will have to look up on any database, such as CINAHL or Medline. Write them down on a piece of paper.
- Now try writing a search statement using the Boolean Operators discussed in Subsection 4.2.1 and the keywords/keyphrases you have identified.

When you have completed the activity return to the next page and read on.

This final section gives you the opportunity to put into practice some of the things you have been learning about in this unit. If you have not already done so, find out what health databases are available to you in your local health, college or professional library. If you are searching the Internet from home here are four free databases that you should be able to use for the next activity. For advice, I strongly suggest you consult your librarian.

- **ENB Healthcare Database search**
  http://enb-search.ulcc.ac.uk/cgi-bin/hcdsearch
  The Health Care Database is a bibliographical database with abstracts for each entry. That is, it acts as a signpost to journal articles and research reports but does not store the full text. You will need to ask at your library for the original sources – journals or reports.

- **PubMed**
  http://www.ncbi.nlm.nih.gov/entrez/query.fcgi
  PubMed, a service of the National Library of Medicine, provides access to over 11 million MEDLINE citations back to the mid-1960s and additional life science journals. PubMed includes links to many sites providing full text articles and other related resources.

- **Electronic Medicines Compendium**
  http://www.emcnet.org.uk/
  This site is free but does require registration. It contains information on generic drugs, products, side effects, dosage and treatment possibilities and is also fully searchable.

- **Current Controlled Trials**
  http://www.biomedcentral.com
  Another site that is free but requires registration and which will provide you with UK clinical trials information. CCT provides access to a searchable database of ongoing UK-funded trials, reports of controlled trials and trial protocols, and links to other online registers of controlled trials.

Remember that navigating your way round the ecology of the Internet will take time but understanding the nature of databases should make it more understandable to you.

Activity 4.8 searching health databases

1 Question: What clinical guidelines are available for the care of people with asthma?
   Task:
   - Identify keyword(s) or keyphrase(s)
   - Write out a search statement using Boolean Operators
   - Test it out on a database.
2 Question: What does clinical governance mean?
   Task:
   - Identify keyword(s) or keyphrase(s)
   - Write out a search statement using Boolean Operators
   - Test it out on a database.

3 Task:
- Think of a subject you would like to research
- Plan, implement and evaluate your search strategies and results. (Refer to Subsection 4.2.2.)

4 Task:

BIOMED provides access to a range of health databases. These include CINAHL, Medline and collections of full text journals. CINAHL is a primary source of bibliographical information for Nursing and Midwifery literature. If you have access to the BIOMED service in your institution, complete **Worksheet 9**. It will enable you to search CINAHL more effectively.

When you have completed the activity return to this page and read on.

Worksheet 9   searching health databases (biomed collection CINAHL)

PART ONE   Biomed (now called Ovid Online) is a collection of important databases provided by Ovid Technologies Inc. . . . (see Section 1.2). To use the service you require an Athens account. To obtain one, talk to the Librarian in your institution/organization.

Accessing BIOMED and starting CINAHL

1 Log on to Windows and start your browser.
2 Log on to Biomed. To do so, in the **Address/Location** box of your browser type http://biomed.niss.ac.uk or http://gateway.ovid.com/athens and then press the **ENTER** key. *A new screen should appear requesting you to enter your Athens username and password.*
3 Type your Athens username and password in the boxes provided then click on the button labelled **Log in**. *Another screen may appear asking you to choose from one of two options.*
4 Click the circle next to **Start a new session**, and then click the **Continue** button. *The screen below should appear giving you the option to choose **one** or up to **five** databases at a time. For the purpose of this lesson we will select only one database to search, so carry out Step 5 below.*
5 Place your pointer on the tab labelled **select a database to search**. If the pointer changes to a hand, then click your mouse button once, otherwise do nothing and move on. The list of databases shown on your screen may be different to that shown in the screenshot below.

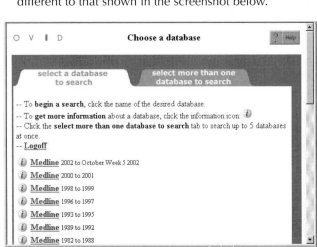

CINAHL is a primary source of bibliographical information for Nursing and Midwifery literature. This worksheet is divided into four parts:

1 Performing a **basic** search
2 Limiting your search
3 Refining your search using **Limit** functions
4 Refining your search using **Combine**.

6 Scroll down the list of databases in the Biomed collection and click on CINAHL **1998 to 2002**. *The screen below should appear.*

Performing a basic search

Comment

You can search for authors or subjects using the database by typing keyword(s) in this white rectangular box. When you click the **Perform Search** button, the computer will then match your keyword(s) to the appropriate subject terms. This so-called mapping facility is useful as it provides some support in selecting search terms.

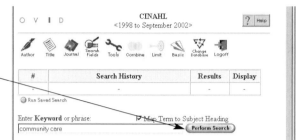

1 Point and click on the white rectangular **Search** box. *A flashing cursor should appear inside that box.*

2 For this activity, type the keyword(s) **community care** (as shown in the screen shot) then . . .

3 Point and click on the **Perform Search** button. *The screen below should appear.*

Comment

A list of subject headings similar to that shown in the screen shot should appear.

Notice that *community care* is not a subject heading. (You may need to scroll down ↓ to see the bottom of the list.) This is because CINAHL is an American database.

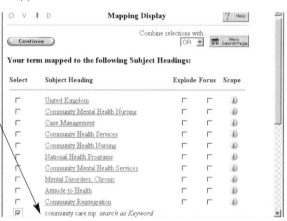

4 Point to the **community care** box and click once. *A tick (as shown in the screenshot) should appear in the white square box.*

5 Point and click on the **Continue** button. (You may need to scroll up ↑ to see it.) *A screen like the one below should appear.*

Comment

Look at your screen under the heading **Search History**. On my visit it shows 403 references on that database for that topic. (Yours may differ.)

Notice the various icons, particularly the Limit function icon. You will need this for the next part.

Also, notice this ⬚ Display ⬚ **Display** button next to the 403.

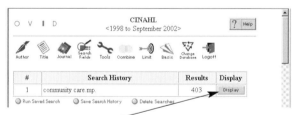

6 Point and click at the command **Display** (or simply scroll down ↓) and you should see a list of references as shown in the screenshot below.

Comment

You are being shown the first 10 of the 403 hits (you may have a different number). This screenshot shows only the first three.

Now you have to decide which reference from the list shown you want to look at. For the purpose of this exercise we will look at record number 1.

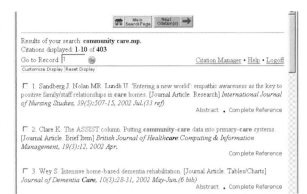

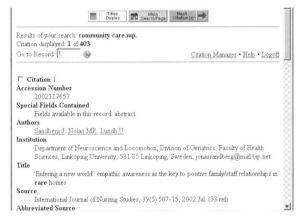

7 Point and click on the command **Complete Reference** (The one next to the record no. 1.) *You should see the screen below appear.*

Comment

This screen shows a long list of headings. These refer to different parts of a published source. Each heading is referred to as a 'field' on a record. The database is composed of lots of these records, each referring to a different published article.

Do not assume everything recorded in this database is available in your library.

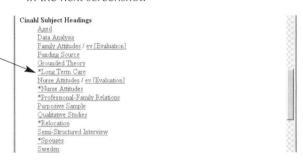

8 Scroll down ↓ the list until you see the CINAHL subject headings as shown in the next screenshot.

Comment

As you can see, some of the subject headings have an asterisk (*) in front of the word(s). These words are what are called the focus of the article, i.e. they tell you what are the most important topics in the article.

```
Cinahl Subject Headings
    Aged
    Data Analysis
    Family Attitudes / ev [Evaluation]
    Funding Source
    Grounded Theory
    *Long Term Care
    Nurse Attitudes / ev [Evaluation]
    *Nurse Attitudes
    *Professional-Family Relations
    Purposive Sample
    Qualitative Studies
    *Relocation
    Semi-Structured Interview
    *Spouses
    Sweden
```

9 To see the abstract for the next citation you simply click on the button marked **Next** located at the bottom of the page. Try it now, if you want.

This brings us to the end of Part One.

The above steps have shown you how to carry out a basic search on CINAHL and browse through the generated list. As CINAHL is an American database, many of the references may not be appropriate or easily accessible. Also, you may not always wish to browse through 403 records (sometimes hundreds more) to find what you want, as this will be time-consuming.

Fortunately there are ways of reducing your search display to a more manageable number. In Part Two, we will refine the search we did in Part One by using limit factors provided by CINAHL database. As you will see, the **Limit** function allows you to limit your search by a number of criteria.

PART TWO *Limiting your search*

1 If you have not already done so, click on the button labelled 🏠 Main Search Page **Main Search Page**. (You may need to scroll up ↑ to find it.) *Your screen should now look like the screenshot below.*

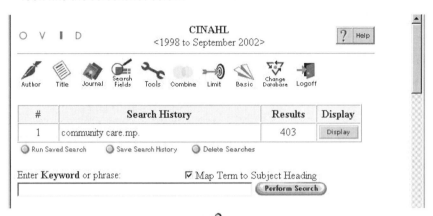

2 Point and click on the **Limit** icon 🎯 *Limit*. *The screen below should appear.*
3 Scroll up ↑ or down ↓ as necessary until you see the display in the screen-shot below.

Comment
We are going to limit our search to UK journals only. This way you may reduce the number of hits and are more likely to display material in more accessible journals. (Remember that this may not be appropriate for all searches.)

ⓘ Age Groups
```
-
Pregnancy
Fetus <Conception to birth>
Newborn Infant <birth to 1 month>
Infant <1 to 23 months>
Preschool Child <2 to 5 years>
```

ⓘ Publication Types
```
-
Abstract
Accreditation
Advice and Referral Website
Algorithm
Anecdote
```

ⓘ Journal Subsets
```
-
African Journals
Allied Health Journals
Alternative Complementary Therapy Journals
Asian Journals
Australian or New Zealand Journals
```

ⓘ Geographic Journal Subsets
```
Australian or New Zealand Journals
Canadian Journals
European Journals
Mexican & Central or South American Jour
UK Journals
US Journals
```

ⓘ Special Interest Category
```
-
Advanced Nursing Practice
Case Management
Chiropractic Care
Critical Care
Dental Care
```

ⓘ Languages
```
-
Afrikaans
Chinese
Dutch
English
Finnish
```

4 Click once inside the window labelled **Geographic Journal Subsets** and drag downwards until you see the **UK Journals**, then click on it to highlight it as illustrated in the screenshot above.
5 Click the **Limit Search** button (**Limit Search**). *The search screen below should appear displaying two searches. The second is UK only. (You may need to scroll up or down to see it.)*

Notice how we have succeeded in reducing our hits from **403** to **274**. If we want to limit the search further still, we can repeat Steps 2 to 3 and add more criteria.

To view your hit point and click on this **Display** Display button and you should see a list showing the first 10 references.

To view any of them repeat Steps 7–9 as shown in Part One.

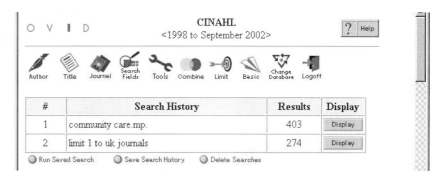

This brings us to the end of Part Two.

In Part Three we will carry out a more advanced search. But, before moving to the next part we need to reset the system. The easiest way is to click on the **Home** button on your Browser's toolbar.

Do this now, and then go to Part Three.

Worksheet 9 continued

PART THREE   *Refining your search*

1 Log on to BIOMED and select CINAHL 1998 to 2002. (For a reminder, refer to Part One Steps 2–6.) *Your screen should now look like the illustration below.*

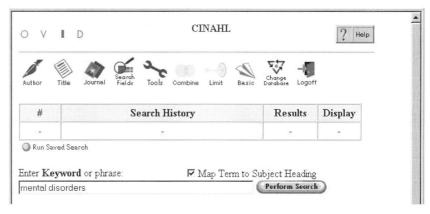

2 In the **Search** box, type the keyword(s) **mental disorders** and then click on the **Perform Search** button. *A Mapping Display screen as shown in the screenshot below should appear.*

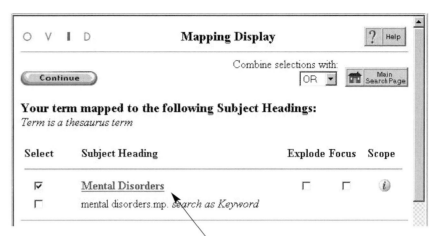

3 Click on the keyphrase **Mental Disorders**. *A Tree display for Mental Disorders like the one below should appear.*

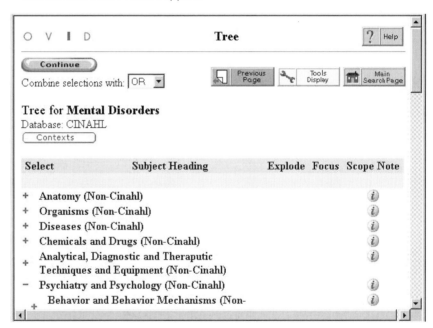

4 Scroll down ↓ and you should see a list of narrower headings associated with **Mental Disorder**.

Comment

Notice how the database has provided you with a list of narrower headings associated with **Mental Disorders**.

Notice also there is a tick in the white box next to the heading **Mental Disorders**. We need to remove it.

− ☑ Mental Disorders (2282)	☐	☐	*i*
+ ☐ Adjustment Disorders (15)	☐	☐	*i*
☐ Mental Disorders, Chronic (221)	☐	☐	*i*
+ ☐ Mental Retardation (990)	☐	☐	*i*
+ ☐ Neurotic Disorders (22)	☐	☐	*i*

5 Point and click the white box next to **Mental Disorders**. *The tick in that box should disappear as shown in the screenshot below.*

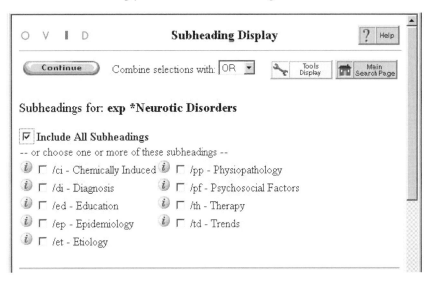

Comment

The **Explode** box ensures that the search will contain not only the term *Neurotic Disorder*, but also all other narrower terms. Thus Explode ensures you capture in your search all associated terms.

The **Focus** box ensures that the search will find only records where the selected terms are the main focus or aspect of the article.

You can use each of these in isolation, or in the same search.

6 Now, do the following:
- Tick the white box on the left of *Neurotic Disorders* to **select** it
- Tick the white box on the right of *Neurotic Disorders* to **explode** your search
- Tick the white box on the far right of *Neurotic Disorders* to **focus** your search.

7 Scroll up ↑ and click on the **Continue** button. *This should move you to the next screen showing you a list of all subheadings.*

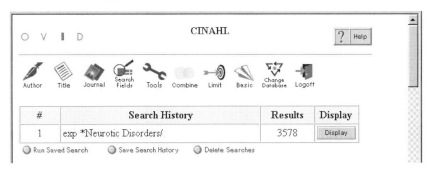

8 Browse down the list of subheadings displayed, and then click the box **Include All Subheadings**. *A tick should appear in it as shown in the screenshot above.*

Comment

After clicking on **Continue** the search will have been completed, displaying how many records on the database are concerned with neurotic disorders where the subject is the main focus of the article. As can be seen in the screenshot on the right, when I carried out my search I hit 3578 records. (You may make a higher or lower hit.)

To browse through all these references would be time consuming. We can reduce the search display to a more manageable number.

9 Scroll up ↑ and click on the **Continue** button. *A screen showing your search history should appear (see screenshot below).*

Exercise 1: Limit your search to UK journals only

Do this now by following Steps 2–5 in Part Two. When you have completed the task, your Search History list should look something like this:

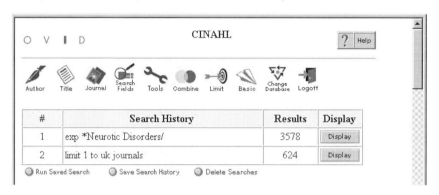

Exercise 2: Limit your search to UK journals and to Adult 19–44 years

Do this now by following Steps 2–5 in Part Two. When you have completed the task, your Search History list should look something like this:

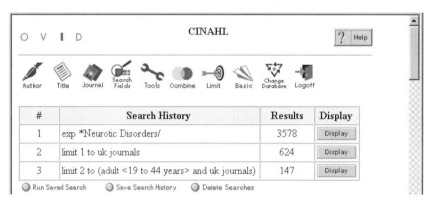

This brings us to the end of Part Three.

We have looked at how we can limit factors to refine search results. In Part Four we will explore another alternative to the Limit option, called Combine search. To use the **Combine** option we need to preserve our current search and carry out a new search.

PART FOUR   *Combine search terms*

1 Use Steps 1–5 under the heading 'Perform a basic search' listed in Part One and carry out a basic search using the keyphrase **community care**. *When you have reached Step 5, your Search History should display four items as shown in the screenshot below.*

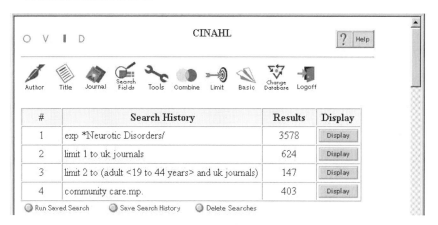

2 Point and click on the **Combine** icon 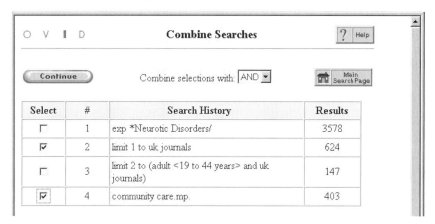. *A Combine Searches screen as shown below should appear.*

3 Point and click in the white square boxes for options 2 and 4. *A tick (as shown in the above illustration) should appear in both boxes.*

4 Click on the **Continue** button (Continue). *A new Search History screen should appear displaying 5 items as shown below.*

Comment

The **Combine** search option has enabled us to reduce the 1027 (624+403) articles to 1 article.

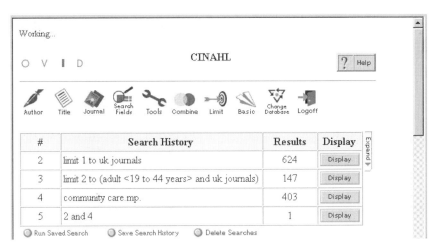

#	Search History	Results	Display
2	limit 1 to uk journals	624	Display
3	limit 2 to (adult <19 to 44 years> and uk journals)	147	Display
4	community care.mp.	403	Display
5	2 and 4	1	Display

5 To view the articles, click on this **Display** command next to 1, and the screen below should appear.

Comment

From here you can:

• Look at the complete reference on the screen
• Print a hard copy
• Save the search or even
• e-mail it to someone or yourself.

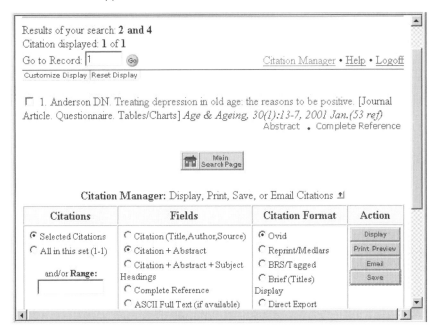

4.3 printing your finds

Once you have located the material you want, you can print the entire document or selected pages.

To print	Do this
Entire document	1 Make sure the printer is Online (i.e. ready for printing).
	2 Point and click on the **Print** icon, located on your browser's toolbar. If you are printing in a computer lab, your request will be placed in a queue until your turn comes.
Selected pages	1 Click on the command **File** on the menubar
	2 Select the **Print** command on the dropdown menu
	3 Type the pages you want printed
	4 Click on the command **OK**.

The Internet is incredibly vast and increases in size daily. The number of sites of interest to health professionals are increasing too. As a beginner to this world of cyberspace you can easily find yourself lost in this unmapped territory of the Internet. Fortunately, there are tools and methods to help you track down what you want for this important research project. *Browsing* and *Searching* are the two main methods of finding information on the net. *Search Engines, Web Directories* and *Information Gateways* are three main types of tools available for searching health, medical and general web sites.

For quality information, Web Directories and Information Gateways are great places to start. However, do remember that they are not comprehensive as they rely on human diligence to maintain them, and it is not humanly possible to keep up with the rapid growth of the web. To conduct a more thorough search, you will have to use one or more of the Internet search engines. Do also remember that some Search Engines provide better searches in different areas of topics. You should try to experiment with them all. The most popular ones tend to get busy in the daytime, so pick your time wisely. A good time is usually when America is asleep.

To make your search more effective, use some of the strategies discussed in this unit. Take time to learn how to use one or two of the search tools available.

Finally, before starting an online search, be clear what it is that you are trying to look for and have a plan.

communicating with other health professionals by e-mail

communicating
with other health
professionals by
e-mail

Even the many nurses who do not at the moment have ready access to the technology can hardly fail to be aware of the existence of the Internet, and the communication possibilities that exist through e-mail.

P. J. Murray (1997)[8]

Lecturer, School of Health and Social Welfare, The Open University, Milton Keynes

Approximately 400 million e-mail messages are sent and received a day over the Internet.

Internet Society

Electronic mail or **e-mail**, is essentially a text system that allows messages to be passed from one user to reach another user who is connected to the Internet or a computer network.

<u>**Electronic mail**</u> or <u>**e-mail**</u> is one of the most popular, hence most used services on the Internet. As a student of health care following a course in a college of higher education or university, after you have registered with your institution's computing services to use their network(s) you will automatically receive an e-mail account. This will not only enable you to send and receive text messages to and from almost anyone in the world who has an e-mail account, but you will also be able to send drawings, software, letters prepared using a wordprocessor, documents or reports compiled from a spreadsheet program, and so on. They will (nearly always) reach their destination within minutes of being sent. Once you have started to use e-mail, you may find that it becomes your preferred method of communication. Health professionals, too, are beginning to recognise the advantages electronic mail has over other forms of sending or receiving written messages. As Information Systems become more evident in hospital trusts, e-mail will become an integral part of it. The knowledge and skills needed to use this electronic system efficiently are not difficult to learn. Many of your fellow students and patients/clients have already mastered the basics. As long as you are prepared to invest some time and effort, you too can enjoy the benefits of this new technology. This unit explains the principles of e-mail, discusses issues associated with this system and looks into how to operate Simeon mail – one of the e-mail programs you are most likely to encounter in educational establishments. Using the same principles you should be able to operate other e-mail programs such as: Outlook Express, Eudora or even Hotmail.

checklist

Below is a checklist of what you can expect to find out in this unit. Read through the statements then tick (✓) the items about which you would like to know more.

I would like to find out more about:

Please now read through the topics you have ticked.

Access code is a unique combination of characters, usually letters or numbers, used in communications as identification for gaining access to a computer. The access code is generally referred to as Username or user ID and password.

E-mail enables you to send and receive messages without the need for either party to put pen to paper. The message can be as long as you want. This relatively new concept in human communication is, in effect, an electronic post office. However, unlike ordinary mail, the address is not a fixed location like a house, but an individual. Hence the individual can access his/her mailbox from any suitable computer terminal anywhere in the world. Like many other users, e-mail is probably going to be the first Internet application you will come into contact with, and may turn out to be the most important for you. Also if you are worried about e-mail messages that arrive while you are *off-line* (i.e. when you are not connected to your service provider's computer), then relax. E-mail will wait for you for a long time.

How?

how does e-mail work?

When you address an e-mail message to someone or vice versa, the message is stored in a central computer in the recipient's electronic mailbox until (s)he checks whether any messages have been received. At that moment the recipient can inspect it, print it out or reply to it. Messages can be left in someone's e-mail box at any time of night or day and will stay there until collected. (Most mail servers only delete messages that remain uncollected when several months have passed by.) Since the central computer stores thousands of electronic mail boxes including your own, this system makes it possible for you to receive and send mail any where in the world using a unique **access code.** This access code ensures that users only get the messages intended for them.

As can be expected even with a good system, there is a downside. E-mail is no exception. For example:

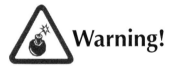

Warning!

downsides of e-mail

- It is against the law to send correspondence such as invoices and writs
- If the line being used is too noisy, e-mail messages can be corrupted
- The facility to respond immediately can encourage hasty, thoughtless replies
- A whiz-kid can break into an e-mail box, though this can be minimized by frequent changing of passwords
- When using the Reply option to respond to an e-mail message, a copy may thoughtlessly go to other people.

Note *For web-based e-mail see Section 5.8.

To use e-mail, you need an e-mail program.* As you can expect, many different programs exist. However, all of them let you do the following:

- Read your incoming mail
- Send new mail
- Reply to messages you receive

- Forward e-mail messages to other people
- Save messages for later
- Print e-mail messages.

5.1.2 e-mail headers

Although different e-mail programs look a little different, the important **headers** are the same. Here is a guide to what these lines mean:

Table 5.1

The important e-mail headers

Header	Description
To:	Here you enter the e-mail address of the recipient.
CC:	If you want others to receive a copy of your e-mail, then type their e-mail addresses in this field.
BCC:	If you want to send the same message to someone else or several other people and you do not want the recipient to know who else is getting a copy, place their addresses in this field instead of the CC: field.
From:	Usually your e-mail software will automatically enter your e-mail address in this field. This tells the recipient who to reply to.
Reply To:	Enter the e-mail address you want replies to be sent to (if different than the From: field).
Subject:	Here you can give your e-mail message a short descriptive label. Although you can leave this field blank, it not advisable to do so. The label you enter will help the recipient to easily identify the message when (s)he looks for this message again a few months later.
Attachment:	Lists the name of any computer files you want to send to the recipient along with the message.
Date:	Time and date message sent is provided automatically by the software.

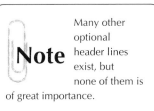

Headers are the lines of text that appear at the beginning of every Internet mail message.

Note Many other optional header lines exist, but none of them is of great importance.

5.2 understanding electronic mail addresses

To send e-mail to someone, you need his or her address and to receive e-mail you need to have an address. The address lets the computer know how to get the e-mail to the right person. Each e-mail address follows an established format and consists of the following basic parts:

- Mailbox name, which is usually the username of your account
- @ (the 'at' symbol) separates the username from the location of the server computer
- Host name or Domain name, which is the address of the Internet Service Provider.

For example, **s.s.chellen@canterbury.ac.uk** is a typical address, where **s.s.chellen** is my mailbox name and **canterbury.ac.uk** is the host name. My mailbox name and the host name are linked by an @ symbol. Hosts are computers that are directly attached to the Internet. Host names have several parts strung together with full stops. Fig. 5.1 shows what each part of an e-mail address means.

Fig. 5.1 The anatomy of an e-mail address

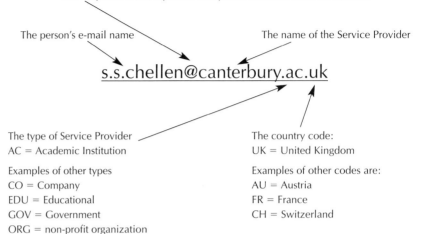

Notice how the whole address is written with no spaces whatsoever and is in lower case.

This @ symbol is the separator to separate the name from the address.

The person's e-mail name

The name of the Service Provider

s.s.chellen@canterbury.ac.uk

The type of Service Provider
AC = Academic Institution

Examples of other types
CO = Company
EDU = Educational
GOV = Government
ORG = non-profit organization

The country code:
UK = United Kingdom

Examples of other codes are:
AU = Austria
FR = France
CH = Switzerland

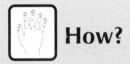

How?

reading e-mail addresses

You may need to verbalize your e-mail address to someone. To avoid sounding like a novice, replace the full stops in the address with the word 'dot' and the @ sign with the word 'at'. Thus, my e-mail address would be pronounced 's *dot* s *dot* chellen at canterbury *dot* ac *dot* uk'.

typing e-mail addresses

Be careful when typing an e-mail address. One typographic mistake will cause the message to come bouncing back to you, never reaching its destination. Ensure that the entire address is written with no spaces.

finding e-mail addresses

By far the most effective way of finding out the e-mail address of a person or organization is to ask them. Where this is not possible, it can be quite a problem because as yet there is no complete 'phone directory' of people's e-mail addresses. Levine *et al.* (2000)[9] suggest the following strategies:

• When you receive an e-mail message from someone, look at the 'From' field, and you should find the address of message author. Copy it down in your e-mail address book.
• Look at the person's business card or stationery, it may list an e-mail address.
• Try using some of the search engines like Yahoo!, AltaVista, DejaNews, and InfoSeek offered on the World Wide Web. You can search on the name of the person or company whose e-mail address you want to find.

Also, all Internet sites that receive e-mail have a person who has the responsibility for sorting out problems with mail. They set up a special e-mail address for this purpose, called 'postmaster'. So if you have a friend you want to e-mail and you know (s)he has an account with a particular service – say Demon Internet – then sending an e-mail to postmaster@demon.co.uk can help you to find her/his e-mail address.

Once you have received your e-mail account from your educational institution, you are ready to start e-mailing anyone in the college or anywhere in the world, provided they have an e-mail account.

In this book I will direct you to a web site where you will find instructions for using Simeon Mail. You should find that once you have learnt how to use this particular mail program, you should have no difficulty applying the principles covered in this book to other e-mail programs. If you have a different e-mail program at your institution (or at home), your own college web site or your service provider may have an online tutorial giving you instructions how to use it.

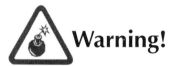
Warning! Always remember that all systems managers have access to user files on their systems, making it possible for them to read other people's e-mail. Whether or not they have the time or inclination to do so is anybody's guess. Most system managers probably would not bother, but it is always possible that some can't help being curious. Also, some institutions may have a monitoring policy. The FBI, too, may set up 'monitoring' sites along the Internet route.

5.3.1 the mechanics of e-mail

Most e-mail programs allow you to do the following:

Send mail	The message is sent to its destination in cyberspace.
Receive mail	You can receive mail addressed to your e-mail account.
Reply	You can reply to e-mail you've received.
Forward	You can send a received e-mail message to another person.
Save	You can save e-mail you've received.
Print	You can print e-mail you've received.
Address book	You can store e-mail addresses.

When you send mail, you need to address it to another e-mail user (by typing the person's e-mail name and address). Make sure you have copied down the e-mail address correctly. Here's an example of an e-mail message from me to a colleague using Outlook Express (which is another e-mail program from Microsoft).

Fig. 5.2 A compose-message window

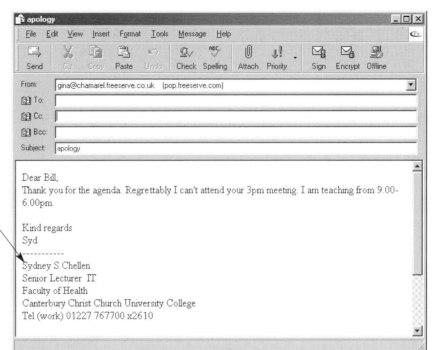

Notice the details in signature at the end of the message? They are usually entered automatically by the e-mail program. (Read Section 5.7.1 below.)

Later on you will have an opportunity to create your signature. First, let's clarify a few things.

Inbox is a term used to describe the box that stores all your incoming mail until it is read.

When an e-mail message has not been delivered, it is 'bounced' back to you, sometimes immediately and other times after a few days. Your bounced message will be in your **Inbox**, along with an automatically generated explanation of what went wrong. If it bounces immediately, this usually means that the address you have typed doesn't exist, or you made a mistake. Occasionally, there may be a problem in delivering the message at the other end. If this is the reason, then try sending the message again. If the problem persists, address a message to the postmaster asking if there's a problem with e-mail delivery and quoting the e-mail address you were trying to send to. For example, if you were trying to send an e-mail to me, say something like this:

I was trying to send an e-mail to:
s.s.chellen@cant.ac.uk
and it bounced.

You can address a message to the postmaster like so:

In the **To**: field, type: **postmaster@cant.ac.uk**
In the **Text area**, you state that your e-mail to *s.s.chellen@cant.ac.uk* has bounced and you would like to know why.

If you have received an e-mail, you can send a reply without having to type the sender's e-mail address and text. For example, let's assume you have received an e-mail and you have opened it into your Viewer window, as shown in the screenshot below.

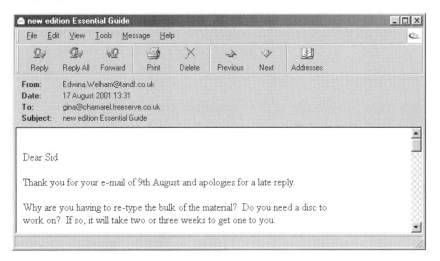

Once you have read the message, to reply to it you just point and click on the **Reply** icon on the program's toolbar. *A Reply window, as shown in the next screenshot, will open up.*

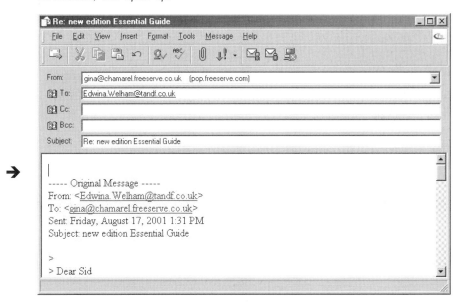

The e-mail program will automatically fill in the address and subject for you. It will also copy the original message into your text area.

A cursor should be flashing where the arrow is pointing. If this not the case, place your pointer there and click the left mouse button.

As you start typing your reply it will push down the original text. When you are ready, click on the **Send** button on the toolbar. Providing there are no errors, after the message has been posted the Reply window should close down.

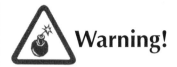

using reply to answer e-mail messages

Be very careful to check all the return addresses Simeon fills in for you – if the mail was addressed to more than one person, you'll be replying to all of them, which may not be what you want. So trim out the addresses you do not want. You can also trim the quoted text as much as you possibly can. It is considered very bad manners to quote someone's entire mail message just to add a one-line reply.

forwarding e-mail and the law

Forwarding e-mail you have received in your Inbox is so easy to do and quite a common practice, but beware as you might be infringing someone's copyright. Steve Gilligan, a learning technology advisor from TLTSN centre at the University of Bangor and a specialist in copyright on the Internet, pointed out during a seminar at the University of Kent that although 'e-mail is something we take for granted these days, all e-mail received from others is subject to copyright protection, i.e. the person who creates an e-mail holds the copyright of that composition'. He added 'if you intend to distribute (i.e. forward) e-mail that you have received, then you should have the permission of that person before doing so'.

Gilligan suggested further that 'under normal conditions an e-mail message will contain information about the origin of the e-mail. This is normally adequate for the purposes of attributing a work to a person. Editing of such e-mail which may mislead people into thinking that, for example, an original idea expressed in someone else's e-mail is in fact coming from you, is an infringement of their copyright'. He added that 'e-mail is subject to the laws of libel and defamation' and concluded that 'e-mail has been successfully used in recent libel cases'. So, be careful what you write and to whom.

If you are ready and have Simeon Mail program installed on your Windows NT workstation or your own computer, carry out the tasks listed in Activity 5.1.

Activity 5.1 using simeon mail

- Get on the net. Type the URL below in your **Address/Location box** of your browser, then press the Enter key. After a few seconds an online tutorial should appear. It contains instructions on how to: **activate Simeon**, **read**, **send**, **reply to**, and **forward** e-mail-messages. Also how to print, save and quit Simeon. Use the on-screen instructions and obtain a printout of the tutorial **SimPart1.htm**

  http://computing-services.cant.ac.uk/title/onlinetutorials/Simeon-Mail/index.htm

- Using the appropriate instructions in the printout, send a short e-mail message to a friend in your college or elsewhere, then close down Simeon. At a later time/date re-start Simeon and if you have received a response, read it, get a printout of the message and then make a reply.

When you have completed the activity return to the next page and read on.

Note When preparing a covering letter to accompany your attached file(s), it is useful to inform your recipient(s) of the kind of document you are attaching. For example, state that it is a document prepared using Word 6.0. This way if your recipients have a problem retrieving the attachment the information given might explain why.

Until recently all e-mail messages could only consist of ASCII text, i.e. the characters you see on your keyboard, with no formatting features like bold, italics, underline, and no drawing or fancy layout. This meant that, if you wanted to design a questionnaire to collect health data for a particular assignment, you were not able to make use of those formatting features mentioned above to enhance presentation. But, with Simeon Mail (and most other modern e-mail programs) you can now 'attach' one or more files to an e-mail message. The attachment can be a word processing file, a chart from a spreadsheet, an image, etc. This is a very powerful facility that you can exploit to your advantage. Now you can use a wordprocessor to prepare your questionnaire. You can lay it out the way you would like it to look, using any formatting features you want. When you are satisfied with your design, you can save it to disk as you would do with any document file. You can also prepare a covering letter to accompany the questionnaire.

When you are ready to send out your questionnaire, you simply attach it to a short e-mail message. In it you should advise your recipients that when they have completed the questionnaire, they should use the **Forward** function to return the e-mail back to you.

While Simeon is sending your e-mail, it will automatically encode the attached file(s), so that it (they) can be sent successfully. When Simeon receives a message with an attachment, it decodes the file and places it on your hard disk. Activity 5.2 will help you send e-mail with attachments.

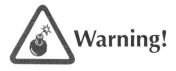

Warning!

attachment problems
In some cases attaching files to e-mail can be tricky, especially when your recipient's e-mail program cannot handle them, either because their program is using a different conversion system. If you know that your software and that of your recipient both use the same system, attaching files is very simple and works well.

Activity 5.2 attaching file(s) to an e-mail message

1 Using your word processor, construct a one-page questionnaire to collect data about the smoking habits of students attending your course, and save it to your hard disk in a directory where you will be able to find it or on a floppy disk.

2 Pay a visit to this web site:

http://computing-services.cant.ac.uk/title/onlinetutorials/Simeon-Mail/index.htm

It contains, among other things, instructions on how to attach a file to an e-mail message. Get a printout of the tutorial: **SimPart2.htm**

3 Now, randomly select the e-mail addresses of the six students on your course who will receive your questionnaire.

4 Using the instructions in **SimPart2.htm**, e-mail the questionnaire to the chosen students as an attachment. Ask them to complete and forward it back to you.

When you have completed the activity return to the next page and read on.

Once you have read your e-mail from your Inbox, it is good practice to either delete it from your provider's mail server or move it to a folder. This is because your provider won't give you unlimited space for e-mail on the server. When your Inbox is full, incoming mail will just bounce back to the sender. You may receive a reminder from the System Manager requesting that you clean your Inbox. Failure to respond to such a request may result in your Inbox being cleaned for you.

The process of deleting or moving e-mail is quite simple. Before you can move an e-mail message, you must have a folder ready to move the e-mail into. This too is quite easy to create, as you will find out by carrying out the tasks in Activity 5.3.

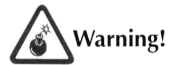

Warning! Be extra careful when deleting messages, because once you have deleted an e-mail message you may not be able to get it back.

Most e-mail programs (including Simeon Mail) enable you to save messages that are similar or deal with the same subject in folders. After you save a message to a folder, you can later call that folder up again and open all the messages in it. Organizing messages in this way can save you valuable time when searching for old messages. In the screenshot below you can see there is a tree with a long list of various folders that I have created for my own use.

Fig. 5.3 Screenshot for Outlook Express folders

List of folders:

1 Inbox
2 Permission
3 Sent items
4 Deleted items
5 Drafts
6 Ecdl
7 Received

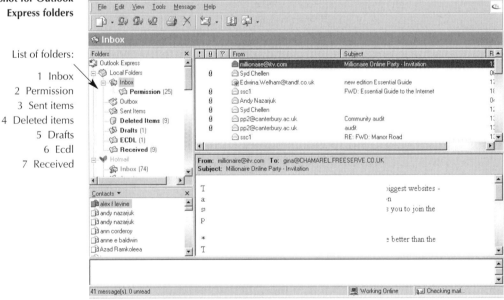

The steps for creating a folder to add to the tree are quite simple. In the next activity you will have an opportunity to create a folder.

Activity 5.3 processing e-mail

Using the instructions in the online tutorial worksheets: **SimPart1** and **SimPart2**, practise the following:

1 Forwarding e-mail messages
2 Saving an e-mail message to a file
3 Printing an e-mail message
4 Deleting and Undeleting e-mail messages
5 Creating a new folder
6 Transferring messages to other folders.

When you have completed the activity return to this page and read on.

5.4 what you need to use e-mail at home

If you would like to send and receive e-mail from the comfort of your home, then you will need a few bits and pieces. You may have a few of them already. The activity below will help you identify your current situation.

Activity 5.4 what do you need?

Here is a list of what you will need to be able to send and receive e-mail from the comfort of your home. Use this checklist to tick (✓) your requirements:

☐ A computer
☐ A *modem* to use with your computer
☐ A telephone line to connect your modem
☐ Communication *software*
☐ Membership of a *service provider* to get on the Internet
☐ An electronic name and address (this will be issued to you by the service provider)
☐ The electronic name and address of the person you are attempting to communicate with.

For more information on the items listed above, please refer to Unit 2, Section 2.3.

5.5 e-mail conventions (netiquette)

There are some simple unwritten rules that you are expected to follow when posting electronic mail messages. These are widely known as netiquette. The rules are equally applicable to postings on bulletin boards, commercial online services and mailing lists. Obeying these rules can make e-mail more useful and effective. Rinaldi12 offers a well-respected guide. Here are a few Dos and Don'ts:

Table 5.2 E-mail netiquette	**Dos**	**Don'ts**
	• Keep your messages short – this makes them quicker to read and more likely to get a reply, especially from busy people.	• Send junk mail – it clogs up the system unnecessarily.
	• Use white space in the message rather than lumping all the text together, and number your topics or create new paragraphs. These make reading easier.	• Use too many words in CAPITAL LETTERS. They are difficult to read and in e-mail this is perceived as yelling, which can provoke an angry response.
	• Be kind to your reader. Punctuate your message properly. Messages that do not use capitals to begin sentences and proper nouns are hard to read.	• Use culturally specific language as a general rule. UK colloquialisms or metaphors may not be understood abroad.
	• Include a snippet of the e-mail you are replying to – it puts your message in context.	• Use words that denigrate someone – libelling someone in an e-mail is an offence.
	• Test your recipient's capability of reading an e-mail attachment before sending one. There is no point in sending an attachment to someone if (s)he cannot access it.	• Assume that your e-mail is confidential; others may be able to read or access your mail.Therefore, refrain from sending or keeping anything that you would mind seeing on the evening news.
	• Keep signatures short and relevant (see Section 5.7.1).	• Reply in heated verbal terms. In e-mail lingo, this is referred to as 'flaming'.
		• Forward someone's private e-mail without his or her permission.

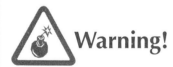 **Warning!**

flaming health professionals

A '*flame*' is an inflammatory criticism directed at another e-mail user. This situation can easily occur with messages sent to newsgroups. A 'flame war' can quickly erupt when other users flame those doing the criticising. Doctors, nurses and other health professionals are sometimes targets for vicious attacks on their personal character and professional reputations by people who are hostile for no apparent reason.

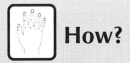

How?

how to cope with e-mail overload

When people find themselves overloaded with e-mail messages, this inevitably leads them to avoid reading their e-mail. This is usually not a useful solution for anyone to adopt as it reduces the benefits of an e-mail system. Here are some strategies that you could use to reduce the problem of overload:

- **Be selective** – (a) When sending e-mail to a number of recipients, decide whether what you are writing is pertinent to all of them. If not, then do not include them on the list of recipients. (b) When you are replying to an e-mail message that has been sent to multiple recipients, the system will usually ask you if you want your reply to go to 'all' recipients. You should only select 'yes' if your response is pertinent to all of them.
- **Good housekeeping** – Delete unwanted e-mail and sort and save useful ones in folders. You could create in-tray folders to help you prioritize your reading and reply of e-mail, e.g. Very urgent, Moderate, Not urgent.
- **Keep to a single idea** – When writing your e-mail, each message should deal with one topic only. This will reduce the length of the message and encourage your reader to read the message.
- **Adopt a business style** – Keep your message business-like. The formality, topics, language, and routing of your e-mail should follow business rules.

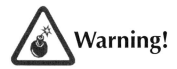

Warning!

composing your e-mail online

When using the network at your college/university, you will normally be composing your e-mail while online. This costs your institution more in phone bills and you may not be able to do anything about that. However, when using your own system at home, remember that you only need to be connected when you are fetching or sending mail. So, check the program you are using and see if it is possible to compose your e-mail message offline.

5.6 using keyboard characters to convey feelings

A bit of humour when sending e-mail can be a nice touch, but making funny remarks on e-mail can quite easily be taken as deep and deadly insults, which could result in a 'flaming' war online.

In face-to-face conversations, or even on the phone, there are all sorts of clues that indicate the real meaning behind words, which help you to determine whether what is being said should be taken affectionately or angrily. On e-mail, this can be difficult but not impossible. Emoticons, otherwise known as 'smileys', are little expressive faces that can be made from standard keyboard characters to convey feelings or to prevent a comment being misunderstood in e-mail messages, newsgroups postings and text-chat. As an example, you may put <s> (for smiling) or <g> (for grinning) at the end of a sentence to say to the reader: 'I am joking'. Here are some recognized smileys:

Table 5.3

Some keyboard characters conveying emotion

Symbol	Meaning
:-)	Indicates a smile or a humorous remark
;-)	Signifies a wink, a joke, or a sarcastic comment
:-(	Indicates a frown or depressing remark
%-)	Expresses confusion.
:-> or >:-)	Signifies a devilish grin
:-||	Indicates you are angry
:-|	Indicates you are not amused
:-&	Indicates you are tongue-tied.

Note When sending e-mail messages, if the e-mail program you are using does not allow the use of bold, italic or underline to emphasize particular words of phrases, you can do it in other ways, e.g. to emphasize text you can surround the word or phrase with asterisks or underline like so (*bold*), (_underscore_).

Note: If you can't make any sense of the above symbols, try turning this page sideways.

By the way, also in common usage are acronyms that came about as a result of Internet users having to compose their e-mail while online and clocking up charges. Although messages can now be composed offline, the use of acronyms has become a part of accepted e-mail style, and you will find them if you get involved with Chat. You can turn just about any phrase into so-called acronyms. Here is a little bundle of them:

Table 5.4

Some so-called 'acronyms' used in e-mail

Symbol	Meaning
AFAIK	As far as I know
BCNU	Be seeing you
BTW	By the way
FAQ	Frequent asked question(s)
FWIW	For what it's worth
FYI	For your information
IMO	In my opinion
IOW	In other words
OAO	Over and out
OTOH	On the other hand
OTT	Over the top
TNX	Thanks.

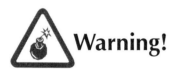 **Warning!**

don't confuse your reader

However interesting, amusing or even useful acronyms and smileys might be, they unfortunately breed a very confusing style of communication. They have been included in this book simply to increase your awareness of their existence. If you must use them, then do so with great caution, for just because you know that IMHO stands for 'In my humble opinion', it doesn't mean that anyone else does.

5.7 other options and issues

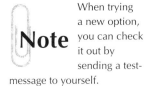

Note When trying a new option, you can check it out by sending a test-message to yourself.

Modern e-mail programs tend to offer more than the basic requirements of composing, sending, receiving and reading. Spending a little time finding what else your e-mail program can do is always time well spent. Here are two options than you ought to investigate when you have a moment or two.

5.7.1 signatures

You can finish off your e-mail messages by adding details about yourself, which are not provided by the mail headers. For example, your name, telephone and fax numbers, the course you are on and a motto. It would be tedious to have to type out all this information every time you compose an e-mail. Signature is an option on one of your program's menus. This option provides a blank space for you to enter whatever text you choose, and this will be automatically added to the end of all the messages you write. Signatures can be fun for a while, but if someone gets a lot of mail messages from you, a signature that takes up a lot of space can soon end up boring. As a rule of thumb, keep your signature as short as possible – in any case it should never be more than four lines. The longer your signature, the lower you are held in esteem by many people on the net.

5.7.2 address books

This is simply a facility, available in most e-mail programs, for you to compile a list of names and e-mail addresses. This way, whenever you need to send someone an e-mail, instead of having to type his or her e-mail address, you can select it from your address book and it will be inserted in the correct place for you. With programs like Simeon, you can also create multiple address books, or you can group addresses into different categories for speedy access. Being able to group addresses is quite useful, e.g. when you need to send the same message to all the members listed in that group, you simply double-click the group name.

Activity 5.5 creating an address book and a signature file

Using the printout from the online tutorial: **SimPart2.htm**, do the following:

- Create an address book in Simeon
- Create a signature file.

5.8 web-based e-mail

An alternative to using a dedicated e-mail program for handling e-mail is web-based mail. You may have heard of **Hotmail** and its rivals like **Excite** and **Yahoo! Mail**. To use one of these web-based mail services, you first need to get on the net and create a free account with one of the service providers. For example if you want to use Hotmail, you can go to http://www.hotmail.com and register for

Note Your university or institution may offer a web-based e-mail facility. For example, if you are a bona fide student at Canterbury Christ Church University College, you should be able to access your college e-mail box from home using their webmail facility.

To access this facility on your home computer do the following:

1 In your web browser's address box, type: http://www.cant.ac.uk the college homepage should appear.
2 Then click on Webmail.
3 To log in, enter your *username* and *password*.

a free account. Or if you prefer Yahoo!, then go to http://mail.yahoo.com to register yourself. Either of them will give you a new e-mail address, a *username* and *password*.

Once you have a web-based mail account, you will be able to read and send e-mail messages almost anywhere in the world using any computer that has Internet connection. If you are away from home, you should find such a computer in a cybercafé or library.

The trouble with web-based mail is that you must be on the net before you can use it. This means splashing out more money on your phone bill or paying to use a PC in a cybercafé. Also, web mail accounts, though useful, are limited because you are only allowed to receive a certain amount of messages. This is almost the opposite of a POP3 mail account (see Section 2.3.5). POP3 (Post Office Protocol, which is currently at its third version), is, more than likely, the type of e-mail account your ISP supplies. If you are with Freeserve, Virgin or Demon Internet, your mail is sent and received using POP3 transfer protocol. To use POP3 you first need to install a software program on your PC and enter all the POP3 settings. Popular POP3 e-mail clients are:

- **Outlook Express** This package works hand-in-hand with the Internet Explorer (IE) browser and when IE was installed on your home system, this would have been installed along with it.
- **Eudora light** You can download this program from http://www.eudora.com

Until recently it was almost impossible to check your POP3 e-mail while you're in a cybercafé. But if you care to use Mail2Web at:

http://www.mail2web.com

you can get the best of both worlds. Mail2Web is a web site that you can use to read, reply and forward messages sent to your POP3 mail account.

Activity 5.6 check your e-mail on the web

Following the steps in **Worksheet 10** access Mail2Web, and then practise reading and replying to a message sent to your home account. (*Caution*: Do not delete any messages that you may need to download in the future.)

When you have completed this activity return to this page and read on.

Worksheet 10

using a web site to read and reply to messages sent to your home account

1 Activate your browser and type the following in the Address/Location box: http://www.mail2web.com, then press the Enter key on your keyboard. The screen below should appear;

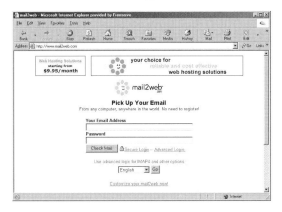

2 Enter your e-mail address and password in the boxes provided. (The password is the one you supply to your Internet Service Provider to collect your mail.)

If Mail2Web can't recognize your e-mail account, click the link labelled 'advanced login page'. The screen below should appear.

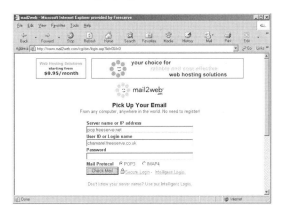

3 Now, enter your *POP3 server name*, your *account name* and your *password* in the boxes provided. Once you have logged in successfully, a screen similar to the one below should appear displaying a list of messages that have arrived in your inbox

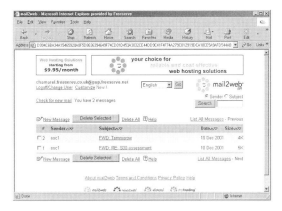

4 To view a message, click the link under the subject column. The e-mail message should appear on your screen.

5 To reply and forward messages, just click the links at the top of the screen. (Screen not shown here.)

6 To attach a file from your PC to a message, just click **Reply** and then use the **Browse** to locate a file.

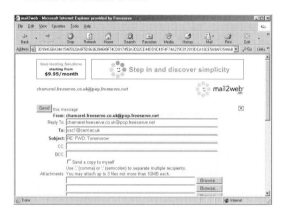

7 When you are ready, click on the **Send** button. The message should go successfully.

5.9 Virus attacks via e-mail

Macro viruses are computer viruses that use an application's own macro programming language to distribute themselves. These macros have the potential to inflict damage to the document or to other computer software. These macro viruses can infect Word files, as well as any other application that uses a programming language.

A virus is a category of *software* which infects *programs* and data files and which replicates itself usually without the user knowing about it. Some appear harmless, simply displaying a message, but others can be very damaging, destroying files and software. Contrary to popular belief, viruses cannot exist in the text of the e-mail message. The danger with e-mail is in file attachments, such as .exe or .com files or MS Office .doc files that can contain a **macro virus**. These file types can all contain viruses and if you open or run one that contains a virus your machine will become infected. So when downloading file attachments always scan them with an up-to-date virus checker. There are a growing number of anti-virus programs that can scan documents within your e-mail program. Most anti-virus software has a web site where you can read about the latest threats and how to deal with them.

Since the explosion of the Internet, the threat of a virus attacking your PC has increased immensely. Although contamination from infected media is still possible, the main threat today comes from e-mail. A virus is most likely to find its way onto your PC by appearing as a bogus file attachment in an e-mail. Having received such an e-mail you may unwittingly infect your PC by double-clicking and opening the bogus file. Not content with infecting your system, usually the virus will scour the contents of your e-mail address book and proceed to pass the infection on to all your friends and contacts contained in it. Using the same sneaky attachment trick, it will attempt to infect them, and then propagate itself through their address books as well. This domino effect can see a virus spread around the world in a very short space of time. While you are never going to be 100 per cent safe from risk of infection, there are some precautions you can take to give yourself a fighting chance against this menace. (Also read Question 3 in the section Twelve Big Questions and Answers.) Here are eight practical steps to fight back against net nasties.

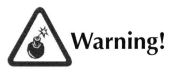 **Warning!**

do not believe everything you read on e-mail

If you receive an e-mail message containing a virus alert, especially those that ask you to 'Copy this message to everyone in your address book', make sure it is not a hoax. You can check to see if it is true on a Virus Page. Useful resources for checking about viruses include:

- McAfee at http://www.mcafee.com
- Stiller Research at http://www.stiller.com
- Symantec Worldwide at http://www.symantec.com
- The Truth about e-mail Viruses http://www.gerlitz.com/virushoax/
- Trend Micro Inc http://www.antivirus.com

Note

Top 3 viruses

Nimda-A Spread via e-mail, this virus can infect Windows 95, 98, Me, NT and 2000. It infects files and attempts to send itself to any e-mail address that it finds.

Sircam-A Comes as an attachment with the same name as the e-mail's subject line. It will alter your Registry and, again, will attempt to forward itself using the names in your address book.

Magistr-A This is a very dangerous virus and can delete files. It can also wipe vital information from a PC's motherboard. It is sent as an attachment and goes under a variety of names.

Grisoft AVG
Grisoft's anti-virus guard package works with Outlook, Outlook Express and Qualcomm's Eudora, and runs in the background. This free package includes lifetime virus definition updates.

8 ways to avoid virus infection

1 **Scan for viruses regularly** – Check your PC regularly for unwanted bugs. Pay a visit to http://www.centralcommand.com/scan.html and you will be able to perform a free scan. Check the E-mails option to scan your mail program for viruses as well.

2 **Install anti virus software** – To give your PC constant protection from viruses you can download a good-quality **free** virus program from http://www.grisoft. com/ This capable package will not only scan your e-mail in both directions, but also provides added reassurance to everyone you send mail to, by adding a footer at the end of every piece of mail stating that the message was checked for virus activity.

3 **Get regular updates** – Virus software that is out of date is at best useless. New viruses come on the scene all the time. Set your PC to remind you of latest updates.

4 **Filter e-mail attachments** – As most viruses are transmitted in the form of an e-mail attachment, you can avoid infection by setting up a mail rule. E-mail programs like Outlook Express can direct e-mails with attachments into their own special folder for closer inspection.

5 **Be on the look out for double file extensions** – You can spot a virus in an attachment by examining the file name. If a file name ends with .VBS (for example message.txt.vbs) you should be suspicious. This is a Visual Basic Script file that may well contain a virus.

6 **Macro viruses** – Word documents can contain viruses hidden away in macros. If you are using Word2000 you can keep one step ahead of infection by setting the security level to high. Do this by clicking on the commands *Tools➔Macro➔Security*, then check the box labelled 'High . . .'.

7 **Take control of your e-mail** – If you are using Outlook Express 6 you can stop viruses sending out messages to the contacts in your address book list by pretending to be you. Do this by clicking on the commands *Tools➔ Options➔Security tab* and check the box labelled 'warn me when other applications try to send mail as me'.

8 **Virus removal tools** – If you suspect that your PC has been infected with a particular virus then pay a visit to this web site: http://www.centralcommand. com/removal_tools.html Here you will find individual tools that will remove thirteen of the most common viruses.

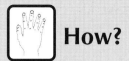

How?

how to determine whether you have a Word macro virus

- Try looking through the various macros for ones that you do not recognize. Some examples of macro virus names are: AAAZAO, AAAZFS, AutoOpen, FileSaveAs, and PayLoad.
- Be suspicious and investigate if your system starts behaving in a strange manner. For example, if you are prompted to enter a password on a file that you know does not contain one or if your document is unexpectedly saved as a template.
- If you see unusual error messages like: '*just to prove another point*'; '*It's time to end all wars*'.
- Unusual changes to your documents; for example, the macro virus may randomly move three words then insert the word 'WAZZU' at random locations.

5.10 handling junk e-mail

A downside of e-mail is unsolicited e-mail. Various companies and individuals gather up e-mail addresses from the discussion forums to compile mailing lists for advertising. There are ways of blocking mail from such sources. One way is to use mail filtering to delete any future mail you receive from that address. With Outlook Express 6 for instance, you can do the following: click on the message to highlight it, click on the word **Message** on the Outlook Express menu bar. Finally, click on **Block Sender**. This will delete the current unwanted mail plus any future mail from this address will be automatically deleted.

summary and conclusion

E-mail is relatively a new form of communication. It can be less expensive and often more informative than a telephone conversation. You can send an e-mail all over the world for very little cost and it will reach its destination in seconds. You can attach spreadsheets, drawings and lots more. Do remember to follow the netiquette and you will find e-mailing a fun way to communicate with other health care users.

joining health
discussion
groups, mailing
lists, etc.

Joining a Mailbase discussion list is an invaluable method for keeping up to date in your area of interest. The lists can range from broad disciplines such as public health and psychiatric nursing, which provide a discussion forum for related issues and highlight new initiatives, developments, conferences, etc., to extremely focused lists such as pupil or acupuncture.

N.J. Howson (1998)[10]
Information Officer, ScHARR – University of Sheffield
e-mail: n.j.howson@sheffield.ac.uk

There are over 25,000 different newsgroups covering every topic you could think of.

Internet Society

A **Newsgroup** is a collection of messages posted by individuals to a news server. A news server is a computer (or program) dedicated to transferring the contents of newsgroups around the net, and to and from your computer. This may be referred to as an NNTP server. These computers are maintained by companies, organizations and individuals, and can host thousands of newsgroups.

Mailing List – This term has two meanings: (a) a list of e-mail addresses to which you can send the same message without making endless copies of it, all with different addresses inserted; and (b) a discussion group similar to newsgroups, but all the messages sent to the group are forwarded to its members by e-mail.

The sheer range of opportunities the Internet offers is beyond belief. In the previous unit we discussed e-mail. Besides exchanging e-mail messages with colleagues or other health professionals you can also join **Newsgroups** – more formally known as Usenet discussion groups. You can find newsgroups on any subject. There are an estimated 28,000 or more newsgroups and hundreds of them are groups concerned with health issues. By joining one or more of these discussion groups you will be able to share your views with other health care students or health professionals. Each newsgroup provides a forum for discussion of issues related to a specialist subject. As a participant you will be able to engage around the clock in group discussions, trade information and ideas with other health care colleagues on the far side of the world. This is a great and fun way to test your thoughts on particular health issues. Lots of patients, too, are using discussion forums. As a health professional you need to be aware of the good and bad points of this medium so you can advise clients.

Another useful and interesting way for people of shared interests to send e-mail messages to each other is via **Mailing Lists**. Mailing lists differ from newsgroups in that a separate copy of the mailing list message is e-mailed to each recipient on the list. By and large mailing lists are more intimate than newsgroups, more specific, usually less riotous, and you can participate regardless of what kind of service provider you have, just as long as you can send and receive e-mail.

In this unit we will uncover some interesting health newsgroups and mailing lists, look at the software you need to access them (both at home and at your institution) and discuss relevant issues.

Below is a checklist of what you can expect to find out in this unit. Read through the statements then tick (✓) the items about which you would like to know more.

I would like to find out more about:

Please now read through the topics you have ticked.

Posting – When you send an e-mail message, the word 'sending' is quite good enough. When you send a message to a newsgroup, it isn't. Instead, for no adequately explained reason, the word 'posting' is used, and the word 'article' is used to describe the message itself.

Usenet news system is a worldwide bulletin board system that allows you to take part in discussions on a wide range of topics and is the main public discussion space on the net.

Oddly enough Newsgroups have very little to do with 'news', as in current events, etc. Newsgroups can be described as a public discussion space on the Net (Russell, 1998).[11] In Unit 5 we looked at e-mail. While e-mail is generally one-to-one communication, newsgroups are one-to-many communication. Discussions take place using e-mail messages (referred to as **postings** or **articles**). Instead of addressing articles to an individual's e-mail address they're addressed to a particular group. Anyone choosing to access this group can read the messages, post replies, initiate new topics of conversation, or even ask questions relating to the subject covered by the group. Some newsgroups are monitored, but most are not. There are no newsgroup membership lists or joining fees.

How?

how do newsgroups work?

Your college or Internet Service Provider (ISP) must have a news server or a link to one. The news server holds articles from thousands of newsgroups that form part of the **Usenet news system**. Once you have set up an account with the news server, you can post messages to a particular group. These messages go to the access provider's server, and are then passed from one server to another (a message takes about a day to go around the world). The messages can then be read by anyone who 'belongs' to that group, and readers can post replies in the same way as they would compose and send e-mail messages. Articles that you post are added to the server's listings almost immediately and are gradually distributed to other news servers around the world.

6.1.1 newsgroup names

Usenet newsgroups are arranged in hierarchies. Here is an example: **comp.sys.ibm.pc**. As you can see, the names begin with words separated by dots. Reading the names from left to right, they begin with a top-level category name and gradually become more specific. In the example above, the newsgroup is part of the **comp** hierarchy, which is generally to do with computers. The **sys** identifies it as being concerned with a specific computer system, rather than (say) a programming language; the **ibm** and the **pc** elements identify it as covering PCs and compatibles.

Although at first glance, there is a bewildering number of newsgroups, almost all newsgroups that you will be interested in can be classified under eight headings as outlined in Table 6.1.

Table 6.1	Hierarchy	Description
Newsgroups of interest to the health professional	Sci	Science-related groups: **sci.med.nursing** (a general forum) **sci.med.occupational** **sci.med.dentistry** **sci.med.pharmacy** **sci.med.diseases.mental**
	Soc	The social groups cover social topics and cultural issues, e.g. **soc.culture.welsh** A very valuable set of *soc* groups is the **soc.support**. This covers a range of mainly long-term and non-life-threatening illnesses, e.g. **soc.support.depression.crisis**; **soc.support.depression.family**; **soc.support.pregnancy.loss** These can be a lifeline for sufferers and their relatives.
	talk	Debates and discussions about controversial topics: **talk.euthanasia** **talk.abortion**
	uk	Most of the Usenet is international in scope. In practice this means that it is overwhelmingly dominated by Americans. Reflecting this, every country outside of the US has its own set of newsgroups. The UK-only groups cover a wide range of subjects. Useful ones to try are: **uk.misc** **uk.sci.med.nursing** **uk.people.support.epilepsy** (an Epilepsy general discussion group).
	misc	Topics that don't fit anywhere else, e.g. items for sale, education, investments and also some with relevance to nursing and health care: **misc.health.therapy.occupational** **misc.health.infertility** **misc.handicap** **misc.health.aids**
	comp	In these groups you will find all sorts of things which are directly related to computers, e.g. **comp.sys.ibm.pc**. This is probably the most useful comp group, where you can find advice from all over the world about using and setting up IBM-compatible PCs.
	news	Groups that deal with the administration of the Usenet news system. New groups are discussed on **news.config**; new groups are announced on **news.announce**. One news group that you should look at is **news.announce.conferences**, which carries a range of conferences.
	rec	The recreation groups cover a wide range of entertainment topics. These groups are usually fairly gentle and helpful, and are a good place for a beginner (generally nobody will be rude to you if you say the wrong thing). Several recreation groups carry review, e.g. **rec.arts.books.reviews**. These are well worth following, since the reviews are by normal Internet users (i.e. probably with similar taste to you).

In addition to the eight hierarchies outlined in Table 6.1, there are several hierarchies that are widely distributed. Table 6.2 shows three examples:

Table 6.2

Other newsgroups which may cover health topics

Hierarchy	Description
Alt	This group is not an official part of the Usenet service, but is still available from almost all service providers. This group covers alternative topics, often of a bizarre and controversial nature: **alt.support.spina-bifida** **alt.education.disabled** **alt.nurse** **alt.society.mental-health** **alt.support.diabetes.kids**
Bionet	Topics of interest to biologists: **bionet.biology.cardiovascular** **bionet.audiology**
K12	Topics of interest to elementary and high school students and teachers
bit	Topics of interest for student nurses and others: **Bit.listserv.snurse-l** **bit.listserv.medforum**

Note

Many groups are moderated. There are strict controls on the creation of newsgroups: a long and involved process of proposal, debate and finally an Internet-wide vote is necessary.

However, in the **alt** hierarchy, almost anyone can set up a group. The sole difference from other hierarchies is that their creators can bypass all the red tape involved in the Usenet process. Much of the pornography is available through alt newsgroups.

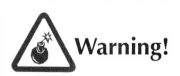

6.1.2 reading articles

Newsreader is the software program you use to access newsgroups, and to read, send and reply to articles.

In order to read articles you need a program called a **newsreader**. There are a number of newsreader programs available and they basically fall into two types. The first type can be described as the *online* newsreader. (If you are planning to use an Internet system at home to read articles, you should avoid this type because to read and post articles you need to be connected, thus clocking up charges.) A better type is the *offline* newsreader.

Warning! Beware, since some offline readers automatically download all the unread articles in your chosen group so that you can read them and compose replies offline. The downside is that in a popular group you may have to wait for hundreds of articles to download, many of which may not be of interest to you. A really good type of offline reader is the one that just downloads the headers of the articles (i.e. the subject line, date, author, and size). Based on this information, you can then select the articles you want to read and reconnect to download your selection.

So, if you have your own Internet system at home and you need a good *offline newsreader*, try Free Agent. This is a popular newsreader and, as the name suggests, it is free. However, if you already have Microsoft Internet Explorer installed on your machine, you will find that the newsreader program is separated and is called Outlook Express (which includes both Mail and News).

Note In <u>Netscape Navigator 3.0</u>, the newsreader is built right in, whereas with <u>NetScape Communicator 4.0</u> the news program is separated and is called <u>NetScape Collabra</u>.

For our next activity I will use the newsreader Outlook Express to show you how to use the **Online Help** to get started with newsgroups. If you're using anything else, for example Agent or NetScape, you will have the same online help available. By the way, do take note that to read news (be it at college or at home), you first need to subscribe to the group or groups that interest you. This does not mean that you have to pay fees, but simply that you need to let your newsreader know which group(s) to download headers from.

Activity 6.1 using your home or college system to read articles

It is assumed that you have Microsoft Outlook Express 6.0 installed on your college Windows NT workstation or on your home system, and that the program is configured for you to be able to join Newsgroups. If this is not the case, the Helpdesk at your institution or your Service Provider should be able to help you.

1 Carry out the steps listed in **Worksheet 11**. They will help you obtain three printouts as follows: How to: (a) *'Subscribe to newsgroups'*, (b) *'Posting messages to newsgroups'* and (c) *'Reply to a newsgroup message'*.
2 When you have obtained all three printouts, use the instructions in the appropriate printout and subscribe to two newsgroups of your choice.

When you have completed the activity return to this page and read on.

If you have successfully carried out the above activity, you should bear in mind that the other subscribers have no way of knowing that you are now a subscriber. All you have done is told your browser what to ask for. You are now ready to fetch and read articles but you are advised not to rush into posting anything. Just spend a few weeks or months snooping on the group(s) you have chosen.

Worksheet 11 using online help to get started with newsgroups

1 Identify the icon labelled **Outlook Express (OE)** and double-click on it. *A dialog box for you to connect to your service provider may appear. Opt for working offline. The OE window should now be clearly visible.*
2 Point and click on the **Help** command on OE menubar. *A submenu should appear.*
3 Click on the key-phrase **'Contents and Index'**. *A dialog box labelled 'Outlook Express Help' as shown below ' should appear.*
4 Click on the section labelled '**Viewing and Posting to Newsgroups**'. *A pick-list of items should appear.*

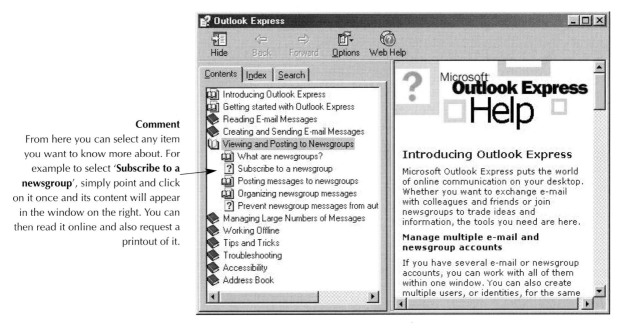

Comment

From here you can select any item you want to know more about. For example to select '**Subscribe to a newsgroup**', simply point and click on it once and its content will appear in the window on the right. You can then read it online and also request a printout of it.

5 Request a printout on the following: **Subscribe to a newsgroup**, **Posting messages to newsgroups**, and **Reply to a newsgroup message**. To print your selection click on **Options** on the toolbar then select **Print**.

The strategy then is for you to be more disciplined in reading articles. First you connect to get the headers, and then you connect again to fetch the bodies of any messages you want to read.

6.1.3 keeping the cost down

By now you would have discovered that there is nothing difficult about fetching and reading articles. You can use Outlook Express, NetScape or even Agent to read articles in two ways:

- If you are not worried about keeping the phone bill down, you can operate any of the above programs in its online mode. This means that your Newsreader is connected to the News server all the time you are reading articles, and collecting them one at a time.
- If you want to keep the phone bill down you can set up your Newsreader to operate offline. This means that your Newsreader will fetch new message headers, collect messages you wish to read, and send any responses you may have set up all in one go. You can then read news offline, while you are not running up the phone bill (reading and replying to articles is the most time-consuming part).

6.1.4 old news

Although the headers are displayed, sometimes you may find that some of the articles are no longer available. This is because old articles have to be deleted to make room for new ones. In popular groups, articles may vanish within a matter of days.

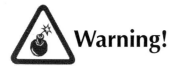

Warning! Occasionally you may come across a message that looks like gibberish. It is possible that the message has been encrypted with a program called ROT13. This program is used to scramble a message to prevent anyone from accidentally reading it, as it may be nasty. The reader can decide whether or not to read it.

6.1.5 newsgroup netiquette

You can learn a lot by just reading articles. However, you can learn even more by getting involved, i.e. by contributing constructively to the discussion. However, before posting anything remember that the e-mail etiquette discussed in Unit 5 Section 5.5, applies even more than ever to articles posted to newsgroups. Newsgroups are quite hot on netiquette. Levine *et al.* (2000)[12] offer the following useful Dos and Don'ts. Most of them have been slightly adapted and reproduced in the Warning box below.

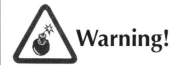

Warning!

1 Don't post a follow-up to the whole group that is intended solely for the author of the original article. Instead reply via e-mail.

2 Don't post a message saying that another message, e.g. a spam ad, is inappropriate. The poster probably knows and doesn't care. Silence is golden.

3 Never criticize someone else's spelling or grammar.

4 If you have to complain about an article, send an e-mail to the post-master at the sender's host.

5 Always make your subject line as meaningful as possible.

6 Be sure that each article is appropriate for the group to which you post it.

7 If you are asking a question, always end your question with a question mark '?'.

8 Don't post a two-line follow-up that quotes an entire 100-line article. Edit out most of the quoted material.

9 Don't cross-post (i.e. post the same article to multiple newsgroups) unless there is a really good reason. Be especially careful when replying to multiple cross-posted messages.

10 Watch out for trolls, i.e. messages calculated to provoke a storm of replies. Remember that not every stupid comment needs a response.

11 Most groups periodically post a list of Frequently Asked Questions (FAQ). Do read FAQ before asking a question as you may find your query has already been answered.

12 As already mentioned, a Usenet Newsgroup is a public forum. Everything you say can be read by anyone, anywhere in the world. Moreover, every word you post is carefully indexed and archived. A simple search on your name displays your e-mail address and a list of every message you have ever posted. So, be careful what personal details you include in your message.

Note Some newsgroups are moderated, generally by unpaid volunteers, which means instead of articles being posted directly as news, they must be posted to a person or program who only posts the article if (s)he or it feels that it's appropriate to the group.

Trying anything for the first time is both exciting and a little bit scary. A completely new news message is called a *posting*. If you reply to someone else's posting, it's called a *follow-up*. You can follow-up to newsgroups, by e-mail to individuals, or both at once.

Here are a few rules that you can follow when you are ready to post your first article. They can make the difference between you enjoying the experience and making you wish you never got involved.

- Pick a newsgroup whose subject is one you know something about.
- Learn as much as you can about the group by reading the FAQ. Many groups post FAQ every few weeks. If you can't see any FAQ, send an e-mail to the group asking if someone could send you one.
- Read the original article and other people's replies to make sure that your point has not already been raised.
- When replying to an article be certain of your facts (be ready to cite references) and make sure that what you have to say is relevant to the topic being discussed.
- Keep your reply short, clear and to the point.
- Pay attention to your spelling and grammar.
- Avoid 'flaming' others with provocative words. Personal attacks in newsgroups can get so out of hand that the whole group descends into what is known on the net as 'flame war'. Don't be the one to start one.
- Read your reply over and over before posting it.

Activity 6.2 posting and follow-ups of articles to newsgroups

Newsgroup messages work just like e-mail: the only difference is that the address you use is the name of a newsgroup, not an e-mail address. You post a newsgroup article just as you would send an e-mail message.

Using the instructions in the printouts '*Posting messages to newsgroups*' and '*Reply to a newsgroup message*' (which you obtained in Activity 6.1):

1 Compose a one-line article and post it to a newsgroup.
2 Select and make a sensible reply to the author of an article.

When you have completed the activity return to this page and read on.

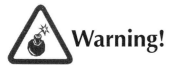

Warning! Attachments are usually not permitted in newsgroups. The charter for **uk.sci.med.nursing** definitely doesn't. (To read the whole charter see www.damien.purplenet.co.uk)

Both Outlook Express and NetScape come with excellent online help. While carrying out Activity 6.1, you would have found the option Help on the

Menubar. Each time you are not sure how to do something, simply click on <u>Help</u> and select '**Contents and Index**'. You'll find lots more information to help you use the many features of your newsreader. Often included are useful tips.

6.1.8 posting header fields

The headers of News postings are very important and can get quite involved. Table 6.3 offers a few suggestions:

Table 6.3
Suggested header fields for News postings

Header fields	Comments
Newsgroups	This contains the newsgroup(s) to which the message will be posted. When putting more than one group in, you should separate the names by commas.
Subject	Whenever you decide to change the subject of a follow-up, it is generally expected that you will include the old subject in brackets. For example a follow-up to a posting called 'UK nursing vacancies' could be 'Nursing vacancies in Kent (was: UK nursing vacancies)'.
e-mail to:	If you put an e-mail address(es) in this field, the message will also be e-mailed to them.
Follow-up to:	If your posting is followed up, this group will be filled in as the default group to post to. So, if you are putting a request about vacancies in the UK to a number of groups, but want all follow-ups to go to alt.nurse, put alt.nurse in the Follow-up To field. If you put 'poster' in this field, follow-ups will be e-mailed to you (the poster).
Distribution	Use this field to limit how far the posting will be passed on to news servers. For example, if your posting is only relevant to UK, put in the distribution field 'uk'.
	Expires: To prevent servers deciding on your behalf when your article expires, put a date in this field.

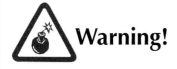

A **thread** is an ongoing topic of conversation in a newsgroup or mailing list. When someone posts a message with a new Subject line they're starting a new thread. Any replies to this message (and replies to replies, and so on) will have the same subject line and continue the thread.

Warning! In a follow-up, check the groups listed very carefully. It's considered bad manners to follow up to inappropriate groups. Also, when replying to an existing thread, you must not change the subject line at all! If just one character is different, newsreaders will regard it as the start of a new thread and won't group it with the other articles in the **thread**, so your reply might be overlooked by the very people who would find it most interesting.

6.1.9 asking for help from newsgroups

If you have got a technical problem, one of the Usenet discussion newsgroups can be the best source of advice. There are a lot of people out there who are willing and able to help. Let's suppose you have a problem you require help with. People are more likely to help if you have taken the trouble of providing a very clear picture. You may find the steps in Fig. 6.1 below worth following.

Fig. 6.1 Eight steps in asking for help from newsgroups

1. Define your problem
2. Choose the appropriate group
3. Check that your question hasn't come up recently
4. Compose your request for help
5. Proof-read it thoroughly
6. Post your message
7. Sit back and wait
8. Say thank you

Let's take a closer look at the above steps.

1. **Define your problem**

   Suppose you have a friend who is in bad shape and needs help. When requesting advice, give as much relevant information as you can. To write to a newsgroup and simply say 'My friend is in bad shape and needs help. What can I do?' is hardly going to get you a useful response. However, if you say something like this: 'I have a friend who has recently suffered some traumatic life events, and could do with some counselling to help get his life back on track . . . Does anyone know where I can get help?' Defining your problem along that line has more chance of getting a reply. So, before putting together your request, gather as much information as possible about your problem. In the example above the problem is with a friend's health. The kind of information you could gather and add to the problem state are: where does he live; is he able to travel to obtain help; has he got a GP or is there any reason why his GP should not be involved? The definition of the problem should be concise yet clear with all relevant details.

2. **Choose the appropriate group**

   It is important that you address your problem to the correct group. In the scenario described previously, any of the following groups may be able to help:

   sci.med.nursing
   soc.suport.depression.crisis
   sci.med.diseases.mental.

3. **Check that your question hasn't come up recently**

   Look through all available postings from the chosen group and if the group keeps a FAQ, check it to see that your problem isn't in it.

4. **Compose your request for help**

   Remember that the people out there are not obliged to help you. A polite request is more likely to produce a positive response.

5. **Proof-read it thoroughly**

   Check all headers for accuracy, in particular your e-mail address. If it is incorrect, any reply you may get will **bounce**.

6. **Post your message**

   When you have done all the above, send your e-mail. Make sure you keep a copy for future reference.

7. **Sit back and wait**

   Once your message is gone, all you can do is to wait. Be patient. Remember that it can take several days before your posting gets round the world.

8. **Say thank you**

   If you have succeeded in obtaining a helpful reply from anyone, show your gratitude by sending a 'thank you' message. It costs nothing and can make people more willing to help you next time.

Bounce means to return undelivered. If you mail a message to a bad address, it bounces back to your mailbox. Conversely, if your e-mail address is erroneous, when people attempt to reply to your message, it bounces back to their mailbox.

Mailing lists differ from newsgroups in that a separate copy of the mailing list message is e-mailed to each recipient on the list.

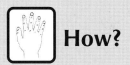

How? A list is set up to discuss a particular topic, and people subscribe to the list. When you send a message to the list, a computer program known as a list server (the actual name may be listserv, listproc, majordomo, or one of several other programs) automatically sends it to all the subscribers of the list. Harmon (1996)[13] reports that there are over 6,500 different mailing lists covering a wide range of topics.

6.2.1 mailing addresses

Each mailing list has two addresses: a *List address* and an *Administrative* or *List Server address*. It is important that you send your messages to the correct one.

1 **List address** – (Almost) anything sent to the list address is re-mailed to all the people on the list. People on the list respond to messages, creating a running conversation. A reviewer scans some lists and (s)he decides which to send out. Use this address for messages you want distributed to all subscribers on the list.

2 **Administrative address** – Direct your message to this address, if you want it to be read only by the owner of the list. You should always use the administrative address when you are requesting something, such as to:

- Subscribe or unsubscribe from the list
- Get information about a list
- Receive a digest version of a list
- Get a list of request commands
- Find all the lists on that system.

List server program is a piece of software on a computer that reads the e-mail you send. For example, if you send an e-mail to subscribe to a list, it will automatically add your e-mail address to its list. For automatic lists, it is important that your e-mail request is constructed in a certain way.

Some lists are maintained manually and others are maintained automatically by a **list server program**. Here is a list of common list server programs:

- **Listserv** – This is a widely used mail server program. It originated in the US and is now used at sites throughout the world by people who have set up discussion lists on their local Internet host computer (Tseng *et al.* 1996).[14]
- **Mailbase** – This is popular in the UK and runs many discussion lists from a single site (at the University of Newcastle Upon Tyne).
- **Majordomo**
- **Listproc**   These are the next three most popular mail servers.
- **Mailserve**

It is often possible to determine if a list is maintained manually or automatically by examining the message header. The administrative address for a list maintained automatically will contain the name of the list server program and, by way of example, might look like this:

Note Some list servers do not care if your administrative request is in upper or lower case, but others do. So be extra careful when typing requests.

- LISTSERV@listserv.acsu.buffalo.edu
- mailbase@mailbase.ac.uk
- majordomo@interaccess.com
- Mailserv@ac.dal.ca

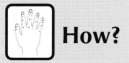

How?

determining an administrative address of a manual list

If you know the list address of a list that is maintained manually, then it is relatively easy to figure out the administrative address. Just add -request to the list address. For example, if the list address is:

midwife@fensende.com

then the administrative address is almost certainly:

midwife-request@fensende.com

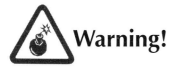

6.2.2 finding a mailing list

Almost any list servers will mail you an index of the mailing lists they support. All you need to do is to send them an e-mail message with the word LIST as the body of the message. Here is an example of what e-mail message to send to the server. Fill the **To** field with the list server administrative address then type the following in the **text area**:

LIST GLOBAL / keyword

Warning!

The keyword is the word to look for in list descriptions and names. If you do not add a keyword, you will get a complete list in your e-mail inbox – about 700K of text. Make sure that your service provider can handle that much mail.

You can also visit the five web sites below, where you should find excellent indexes and search options to mailing lists:

* http://www.liszt.com
* http://www.reference.com/
* http://www.topica.com/
* http://www.lsoft.com/catalist.html
* http://www.jiscmail.ac.uk

To get you started, Table 6.4 offers the administrative addresses of a few mailing lists related to specific topics. For a more comprehensive list, visit any one of the web sites listed above.

Table 6.4
Addresses for mailing lists related to specific topics

List name With brief description where appropriate	To subscribe: Type this address in the field labelled *To:*	Type this message in the *Text* area
ADDICT-L	listserv@kentvm.kent.edu	subscribe addict-1 [YourFirstName] [YourLastName]
AROMA-TRIALS (Related to aromatherapy)	mailbase@mailbase.ac.uk	subscribe AROMA-TRIALS [YourFirstName] [YourLastName]
CANCER-L	listserv@wvnvm.wvnet.edu	subscribe CANCER-L [YourFirstName] [YourLastName]
CHINs (Community Health Information Networks)	chins-request@chin.net	subscribe chins
Rogers Theories	mailbase@mailbase.ac.uk	JOIN nurse-rogers [YourFirstName] [YourLastName]
PSYCHIATRIC-NURSING (Psychiatric Nursing Discussion Groups)	mailbase@mailbase.ac.uk	Join Psychiatric-Nursing [YourFirstName] [YourLastName]
CLINICAL FORENSIC NURSING	listserv@ulkyvm.louisville.edu	subscribe ClForNsg [YourFirstName] [YourLastName]
CRITCARE	requests@critical-care.co.uk	subscribe critcare
EMERGENCY NURSING	listserv@itssrv1.ucsf.edu	subscribe Em-Nsg-L [YourFirstName] [YourLastName]
HCARENURS (Home Health Nursing Mailing Lists)	majordomo@po.cwru.edu	subscribe HcareNurs [YourE-mailAddress]
HOSPICE	majordomo@po.cwru.edu	subscribe hospice [YourE-mailAddress]
NP-STUDENTS (Nurse Practitioner Listserver)	majordomo@wizards.net	subscribe np-students [Your E-mail Address]
PNN-L (This is a discussion group group for nurse practitioners interested in health promotion, prevention and education)	majordomo@interaccess.com	subscribe PNN-L [YourE-mailAddress]
PSYNURSE	listserv@sjuvm.stjohns.edu	subscribe PSYNURSE [YourFirstName] [YourLastName]
MIDWIFE	midwife-request@fensende.com	Subscribe
AIDS	majordomo@wubios.wustl.edu	Subscribe aids L [YourE-mailAddress]
AUTISM	LISTSERV@utkvm.utk.edu	Subscribe ANI-L [YourFirstName] [YourLastName]
CLICK4HP (Health Promotion)	listserv@yorku.ca	Subscribe click4hp [YourFirstName] [YourLastName]

List name With brief description where appropriate	To subscribe: Type this address in the field labelled *To:*	Type this message in the *Text* area
DEVELOPMENTAL DISABILITIES	LISTSERV@RELAY.ADP.WISC.EDU	Subscribe DDHEALTH
GROUP PSYCHOTHERAPY	listserv@natcom.com	Subscribe Group-Psychotherapy
NURSERES (Nurses Research List)	listserv@listserv.kent.edu	Subscribe NurseRES [YourFirstName] [YourLastName]
NURSE-UK (for nurses interested in UK issues)	majordomo@bham.ac.uk	Subscribe nurse-uk
PEDIATRIC-PAIN	mailserv@ac.dal.ca	Subscribe Pediatric-Pain [YourFirstName] [YourLastName]
DRUGABUS	listserv@umab.umd.edu	sub drugabus [YourFirstName] [YourLastName]
NURSENET (discourse about diverse nursing issues)	listserv@listserv.utoronto.ca	Sub NurseNet [YourFirstName] [YourLastName]
NURSGRAD (This is for the discussion of topics related to graduate nursing education)	listserv@ulkyvm.louisville.edu	Sub NURSGRAD
SNURSE-L (For undergraduate nursing students)	LISTSERV@listserv.acsu.buffalo.edu	Sub Snurse-l [YourFirstName] [YourLastName]
CANCER-NURSING-ALLIANCE	mailbase@mailbase.ac.uk	join cancer-nursing-alliance [YourFirstName] [YourLastName]
HEALTH-SERVICES-RESEARCH	mailbase@mailbase.ac.uk	join health-services-research [YourFirstName] [YourLastName]
PAEDIATRIC-NURSING-FORUM	mailbase@mailbase.ac.uk	Join paediatric-nursing-forum [YourFirstName] [YourLastName]

6.2.3 getting on and off a mailing list

Note Most mailing lists are open, meaning that anyone can send a message to the list. Some lists, however, are closed and accept messages only from subscribers. Other lists accept members by invitation only.

Remember that the way you get on or off a mailing list – subscribing or unsubscribing – depends on how the list is maintained, i.e. whether it is maintained manually or automatically.

For lists that are maintained manually, simply send an e-mail message (like '*please add me to the midwife list*' or '*please remove me from the midwife list*') and send it to the administrative address of that mailing list. The message is read by humans, so no fixed form is required. Do make sure you include your real name.

To subscribe or unsubscribe to a list maintained automatically, you must follow a specific format. Unfortunately, the format that needs to be used to make requests differs slightly from server to server. Generally, to join a list you send an e-mail message to its administrative address with nothing written in the *cc*, *bcc* or *subject fields*, but giving the following basic information in the text area: *List name*, *your first name*, and *your last name*. Suppose we wanted to subscribe to 'ADDICT-L' (see Fig. 6.2 below):

Fig. 6.2 Setting up a subscription to a mailing list

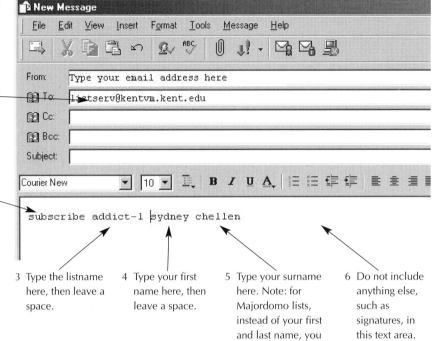

1 Type the administrative address here, as shown in the example.

2 Type this keyword here, then leave a space. Note:
- For Mailbase lists, you need to replace this keyword 'subscribe' with JOIN (to subscribe) or LEAVE (to unsubscribe)
- In some cases the first letter of the keyword or the whole word must be in upper case.

3 Type the listname here, then leave a space.

4 Type your first name here, then leave a space.

5 Type your surname here. Note: for Majordomo lists, instead of your first and last name, you need to insert your full e-mail address.

6 Do not include anything else, such as signatures, in this text area.

Most, if not all, of the list servers listed in Table 6.4 above will respond to the keyword 'UNSUBscribe' so that you can remove yourself from a list. Send this request to the respective listserver *administrative address*, not the *list address*. For example, for ADDICT-L, address an e-mail to listserv@kentvm.kent.edu and in the text area type: **Unsubscribe addict-l**

When you subscribe to any of the lists mentioned, you will generally be sent a welcome message with instructions for posting to the list, unsubscribing, etc. Save this message, you will need it later. If you need additional information on how to subscribe to mailing lists you can pay a visit to:

http://www.dundee.ac.uk/

Note Generally you don't need to include your e-mail address because it is automatically included as your message's return address.

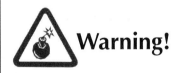

Warning!

- When subscribing to a list, make sure you send your e-mail message from the computer to which you want list messages mailed. This is important, because the administrator of the list uses your message's return address as the address (s)he adds to the mailing list.
- Do not subscribe to too many lists at the same time, especially popular lists, as they generate a huge amount of e-mail. You do not want to drown yourself in a deluge of e-mail.
- When you know you won't be able to download your e-mail, for example when going on leave, consider unsubscribing from your mailing lists for that period, unless you want to be faced with an overwhelming barrage of e-mail when you log on after your break.

Activity 6.3   subscribing to a mailing list

Using the information given above, select and subscribe to a mailing list. For additional information, I suggest you visit NMAP at: http://nmap.ac.uk/ (a gateway to evaluated, quality Internet resources in Nursing, Midwifery and allied health professions, aimed at students, researchers, academics and practitioners) and search for 'emails lists'.

When you have completed the activity return to this page and read on.

6.2.4 receiving mailing list messages

As soon as you have joined a list, you will automatically receive all messages from the list along with the rest of your e-mail. As some lists are available in digest form with all the day's messages combined in a table of contents, you may prefer this digest format. To get the digest form you can send an e-mail message to the list's administrative address with the following lines in the body of the message:

Table 6.5
To receive mailing list messages in digest format

For list server	Type this request in the body of your e-mail message
Listproc	Set <listname> mail digest
LISTSERV	Set <listname> digest
Majordomo	Subscribe <listname> digest, Unsubscribe <listname>

To undo the digest request

Listproc	Set <listname> mail ack
LISTSERV	Set <listname> mail
Majordomo	Unsubscribe <listname> digest, Subscribe <listname>

6.2.5 sending messages to a mailing list

To send messages to a list that you have subscribed to, you will need to know which computer runs that list (i.e. its *list* address, which should be in the details that are returned to you upon subscription). Your message is then automatically distributed to the list's members.

As some lists are screened by a reviewer before being sent off, your message may take a day or two before reaching the members. Good mail servers usually send you copies of your own messages to confirm that they were received. If you have subscribed with Listproc or LISTSERV, you can tell them not to send you copies of your own messages by sending the following message to the administrative address:

Table 6.6
To avoid receiving copies of your own messages

For list server	Type this request in the body of your e-mail message
Listproc	Set <listname> mail noack
LISTSERV	Set <listname> noack

To resume receiving copies of your own messages

Listproc	Set <listname> mail ack
LISTSERV	Set <listname> ack

Note In the <listname> you need to type the actual name of the list without the smaller (<) or greater (>) signs.

After subscribing to a mailing list, there are a few important or desirable requests that you may wish to make. Such as:

- The location of their archive of past messages
- Obtaining a list of all the people who subscribe to the list
- Not wanting your name to be given out to other members.

Here is how to request some of them.

 How?

locating archives of past messages

Send an e-mail to the administrative address. In the body of the e-mail you should type:

INDEX <*listname*>

For example, if you subscribe to the Sociology-Midwifery Mailbase List, you can send an e-mail to:

Mailbase@mailbase.ac.uk

with the following in the body of the e-mail:

INDEX sociology-midwifery

 How?

obtaining a list of subscribers

Send an e-mail to the administrative address. In the body of the e-mail you should type the appropriate keyword for that list server:

For list server	Type this request in the body of the e-mail message
Listproc	Recipients <listname>
LISTSERV	Review <listname> by name f=mail
Mailbase	Review <listname>
Mailserve	Send <listname>
Majordomo	Who <listname>

 How?

concealing your name

Listproc and LISTSERV won't give your name out by the proceeding process if you send an e-mail to the administrative address.

For list server	Type this request in the body of the e-mail message
Listproc	Set <listname> conceal yes
LISTSERV	Set <listname> conceal

To unconceal yourself

Listproc	Set <listname> conceal no
LISTSERV	Set <listname> noconceal

List servers can do many more tricks. If you want a list of those tricks address an e-mail to:

LISTSERV@ubvm.cc.buffalo.edu

and in the body of the e-mail type:

Get mailser cmd nettrain f=mail

6.3 starting an internet relay chat (irc)

IRC provides real-time conferencing over the Internet. It can be useful for talking to health care professionals or students on other continents. However, IRC is not available on all systems, as it tends to use more resources than most system administrators care to devote to it. So, you may find that you cannot use your college network to hold live conversations with others. However, if you have the appropriate system at home you certainly can connect and use this service.

IRC has been described as the CB radio of the net and it is one of those services that you either love or hate (Russell, 1998).[15] You can join one or more 'channels' (i.e. chat rooms) and chat real-time to other health care professionals or health care students – who can be all over the world. The experience is immediate and can bond you with other people quite quickly.

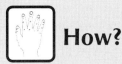

How?

With IRC you hold live conversations with others by typing on your keyboard. You type a line or two of text into a small window and press the **Enter** key, and the text is almost instantly visible to everyone else taking part. They can respond by typing their own messages, and you'll almost instantly see their responses on your screen. There are now IRC client programs appearing on the market, which allow a bit more of the point-and-click approach.

Note In the Internet world, **Chatting** and **Talking** are not the same things. But one thing they have in common is their immediacy.

Chatting usually takes place in a chat room, which may contain just two or three people, or as many as fifty. Sometimes, no one seems to talk at all. Sometimes two or three conversations are going on between little groups of people, with all messages appearing in the same window, and things can get a bit confusing. Although there may be several people in the room, many are just 'listening' rather than joining in.

Talking is a little different. Although the method of sending messages to and fro is the same, 'talk' usually takes place between just two people, and in a more structured way.

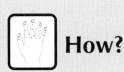

How?

Using a talk program, you'd usually enter the e-mail address of the person you want to talk to, and if that person is online, the conversation begins.

To cloud the issue a bit, *chat programs* also allow two people to enter a private room and 'talk', and many talk programs will allow more people to join in with your conversation if you allow them to enter. This has somewhat smeared the boundary between chat and talk. To complicate things even more, with the recent arrival of Voice on the Net (VON), you can talk to others using microphones (see Section 6.4).

6.3.1 connecting to IRC

The Internet Relay Chat, is the Internet's own chat system. You can connect to it using *Telnet* (for more information see Unit 7, Section 7.4). If you are a beginner you may find that a better approach is to use a piece of software called mIRC. You can download a copy of this program from http://www.mirc.co.uk

To use IRC you first have to connect to your nearest IRC server. There are IRC servers all over the Internet and you can connect to whichever IRC server you want, but you'll get better performance if you choose one close to you. In the UK, the best one to use is **irc.demon.co.uk** run by Demon Internet. If you have a computer system at home with the Internet facility, then do the activity below – it will help you get started.

Activity 6.4 using mIRC to chat and talk

Unless you've already got mIRC installed on your machine, before doing this activity you must first get on the Net, download and install mIRC on your computer. Then, use the program to get connected to an IRC server so that you can start a live conversation.

When you have completed the activity return to this page and read on.
If you don't want to or can't do this activity, read on now.

6.3.2 some irc commands

There are a huge number of commands that you can master and put to use. The mIRC program even includes a general IRC help-file, which explains how they work. A selected few are listed in Table 6.7 to get you started.

It is very easy to use the commands listed previously. Here is a quick example. Suppose you have been holding a chat. You have decided to stop and feel the need to explain why. You can enter this command

/quit Got a lecture to attend. See you tomorrow.

	Type this	To do this
Table 6.7	**/help**	Get general help on IRC
A selection of useful IRC commands	**/list**	List all the channels available on the server you are connected to
	/list -min n	List all the channels with at least *n* people in them (replace *n* with a figure)
	/join #channel	Enter a channel. Replace channel with the name of your chosen channel
	/leave #channel	Leave the specified channel (or the channel in the current window if no channel is specified)
	/quit message	Finish your IRC session and display a message to the channel if you enter one (see below)
	/away message	Tell other occupants you're temporarily away from your computer, giving a message
	/away	With no message, means that you're no longer away
	/whois nickname	Get information about the specified nickname in the main window

Remember that all commands start with a forward slash.

6.4 hearing your voice on the net

Voice on the Net (VON) is the latest addition to the net. It is the Internet equivalent to the telephone. You can hold live conversations with anyone in the world, provided the person is online and has their VON software running.

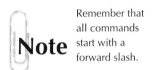

How? You start the VON program, choose the e-mail address of the person you want to converse with, and as soon as the link is established you can start speaking into a microphone. You will hear their responses through your speakers or a headset.

This is a very cost-effective way of holding a conversation with someone far away. Suppose you are in the UK and want to converse with someone in New Zealand. You simply dial into your local access provider, paying only a local telephone call, even though you are speaking to someone abroad. Apart from this, you can send computer files back and forth, hold conferences, or even use a whiteboard to draw sketches and diagrams. However, as both you and the person you are calling must be online, both of you will pay telephone charges. Despite this downside, the combined cost could still amount to less than 10% of a conventional international call charge. Some recent systems allow you to dial someone's telephone number rather than e-mail address, making it possible to make these cheap international calls to someone who doesn't even have their own Internet account.

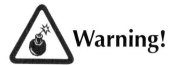

| **Warning!** | Currently, you must be using the same VON program as the other person you want to converse with. If you have several people you want to talk to, you may need to have several different VON programs installed on your computer. Fortunately, some VON programs are free. The situation is bound to change. |

Activity 6.5 checklist of hardware specifications

A **full-duplex** card can record your voice while playing the incoming voice. This enables both of you to talk at the same time (ideal for discussions). With half-duplex you can either talk or listen, but not both.

VON programs have some definite hardware specifications. Use this checklist to tick (✓) your requirements.

☐ A sound card (preferably a **full-duplex** card)
☐ A fairly fast computer, e.g. with a Pentium chip
☐ 8Mb RAM or more
☐ A microphone and speakers plugged into your sound card
☐ A modem 28.8Kbps or higher connected to a phone line
☐ VON software.

6.4.1 a selection of von programs

There is a wide selection of VON programs to choose from. Here is a short list:

1 Internet Phone – A VON program that you will need to pay for, otherwise your talk time will be limited. You can obtain and register an evaluation copy at http://www.vocaltec.com
2 NetMeeting – A Microsoft VON program. You can download a free copy from http://www.microsoft.com/netmeeting
3 Web Phone – A very stylish VON program. For an evaluation copy visit http://www.itelco.com

summary and conclusion

Newsgroups form an important part of the Internet. Getting involved in these can be an interesting and informative way of trading information. A more personal manner of communicating is with mailing lists. Both of those methods can prove to be useful sources of information and the people involved in the newsgroups may be able to solve your problems. If you want a faster medium then try IRCs. These can also prove useful but also quite expensive if done from a home PC.

the gateway to free health and medical resources

I used to have to drive 30 miles to get to my college library, only to discover that the books I need are out or unavailable. Now, from the comfort of my own home I can telnet into my library computer, browse through their catalogues and order the books I want. All with a few clicks of my mouse.

A part-time BSc student

FTP stands for File Transfer Protocol. It is a method of transferring files from one computer to another over the net.

Archie is an older system that was and can still be used to find files that are located on the FTP sites.

Gopher is an older system that lets you find text information by using menus.

Telnet is a system that lets you connect from your computer to another across the Internet and use it as if you were directly connected to that computer. A slightly different version of Telnet, developed by IBM, is known as tn3270.

Although e-mail and the web will probably meet most of your needs, there are additional tools that you will hear mentioned which can help you use your browser more effectively. They were around long before the World Wide Web started dominating the Internet.

Four of these are **FTP**, **Archie**, **Gopher** and **Telnet**. The functions of many of these tools are now performed by web browsers like NetScape Navigator or Microsoft Internet Explorer. However, there may be occasions when it is necessary for you to use these tools directly to gain access to all those millions of computers around the world. For example, you may become aware of statistics that support a project you are completing, a computer program that can help you perform your health data analysis, or documents that offer a bibliography for a course assignment. With the right privilege you can grab these files and transfer them to your computer free of charge. Or you may need to quickly search a computerized library catalogue to find available material to complete a project, but do not wish to trot from library to library.

In this unit, the four tools mentioned above will be discussed. It includes explanation on how to use them to find what you want, and where appropriate how to download your find to your hard disk.

checklist

Below is a checklist of what you can expect to find out in this unit. Read through the statements then tick (✓) the items about which you would like to know more.

I would like to find out more about:

Please now read through the topics you have ticked.

7.1 ftp (file transfer protocol) - what is it?

Links are hypertext, identifiable by being underlined and a different colour from the ordinary text around it. Links can take you to other documents or other parts of the same document. On the web, links can appear as text or pictures.

Note FTP sites are usually prefixed with **ftp://** . . . The only exception is when the name of the computer starts with 'ftp', but in these cases you can still use the prefix if you prefer.

FTP stands for File Transfer Protocol. It is a method of transferring files from one computer to another over the Net. It works in a similar way to File Manager (on Windows 3.1 and NT) and Windows Explorer on Windows 95/98/2000. While with File Manager or Windows Explorer you can open directories, browse around and copy any file to another directory on your hard disk or floppy disk, with FTP you can copy files from another computer to your own or vice versa.

While completing Units 2, 3 and 4 you have already made some use of FTP without perhaps realizing it. You may recall while surveying web pages you have been clicking on **links**. These links were letting you download files. Some of these files were stored on web servers and others on FTP servers. Next time you surf the net, and you come to a link, simply rest your mouse-pointer on the link and look at your browser's status-bar. If the link is pointing to an FTP site, you will see the address starts with **ftp://**

The addresses (URLs) of FTP sites look almost like web addresses. They begin with the type of server (computer) and continue with the directory path to the specific file. Here is a quick comparison of the two URLs. Notice that one starts with *http://* and the other starts with *ftp://*

A web URL: http://www.diabetic.org.uk/index.htm

An ftp URL: ftp://ftp.liv.ac.uk/pub/epidemic/

Before exploring how to get into ftp sites, let's first clarify the difference between private and anonymous sites.

7.1.1 private vs. anonymous sites

Some FTP sites are called **anonymous** because the system does not need to find out who you are before letting you in. You can log in to these sites by entering the word *anonymous* for username and for password you enter your e-mail address or simply type the word *guess*.

Some FTP sites hold confidential files and therefore only users with special privileges can access them. They are known as private FTP sites. Many other sites, known as **anonymous** FTP sites, give free access to all their files. However, some of these anonymous sites may have only their top-level directory called pub or public which contain non-confidential files. In that case, the public can access only these non-confidential files.

Whether you are trying to access a private or anonymous site you will need a username and a password to log in, just as you do when you connect to your service provider's system.

If you have a special account with privileges to access confidential files on a private or anonymous site, when you log in the computer will recognise who you are by your username and password. In this unit we are going to concern ourselves with access to anonymous sites that are open to the public.

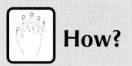

How?

how to get access to FTP sites

To get access to FTP sites you simply connect your computer to an FTP server – an Internet host computer that stores files for transfer. To make this connection you can use one of the following:

- Your browser,
- A real FTP program, or
- Your e-mail program.

In the next three sections, all the above will be discussed.

7.1.2 accessing ftp sites

You can use Microsoft Internet Explorer, NetScape Navigator (or any other browsers) to access non-confidential files at any anonymous FTP sites. As the two browsers mentioned above are so sophisticated, you won't be prompted to enter anything. The browser will handle everything automatically for you. The activity below will show you how easy it is to use Internet Explorer (or NetScape Navigator) to access a file on an FTP site.

Activity 7.1 using your browser to access ftp sites

Let's suppose you're looking for the *Liverpool School of Tropical Medicine Meningitis Epidemic Case Study*. You have been told that the file is called **epidemic** and it is located at this URL: ftp://ftp.liv.ac.uk/pub/epidemic/

Using the knowledge and skills you have or have acquired from previous units in this book, go and get this file. (*Clue*: log on to Windows and start your browser. Type the URL in the **Location/Address** box, then press the Return key. Provided there is no problem, the requested page should appear on your screen.)

When you have completed the activity return to this page and read on.

The above activity was not too difficult, I hope. You may have noticed that it was no different to searching for a known file on the web, except that you had to go to an ftp site to locate it. The next section will discuss the second method of obtaining files from ftp sites.

As you begin to get more acquainted with the Internet, you may want more control over the file transfer process – especially when later on you create your own web site and you want to copy files to your access provider's web server. In this case, you would find a 'real' FTP program more user-friendly, and sometimes it will connect to an FTP site faster than a browser can. A dedicated FTP program also gives you more information about the progress of downloads from FTP sites than a browser does. There are several ftp programs that you can use. Here are two of the best FTP programs around currently:

- **WS_FTP LE for Windows** – A very popular program. You can find the fully-fledged WS_FTP Professional including updates at this web site: http://www.ipswitch.com
- **FTP Explorer** – A nice little program designed for Windows95 and later. For a version of it look at http://www.ftpx.com

When you use FTP programs like those described above, you simply click on the label **Anonymous** and all necessary details will be entered for you. You may find that your college/university has one of these FTP programs – or a similar one – already installed on the network.

If you have Internet access at home, you may wish to install it on your system. To do this, pay a visit to the web sites given above and grab a copy of WS_FTP or FTP Explorer. You should find on-screen instruction on how to download the program. Installing WS_FTP is simplicity itself. Activity 7.2 offers some assistance.

Activity 7.2 using a dedicated ftp program to access ftp sites

You only need to carry out this activity if you would like to use one of the two FTP programs mentioned previously, on your home system, with a view to surfing FTP sites.

- Log on to the Internet (using your home or college system) and enter the URL http://www.ipswitch.com in the **Address/Location** box of your browser. Once you are at the web site containing the WS_FTP program, follow the on-screen instructions and download it to a floppy disk.
- Following the instructions in **Worksheet 12**, create a 'Session Profile' that will connect you to an FTP site in WS_FTP.
- Now, using the WS_FTP program, see if you can replicate the activity in Section 7.1.

When you have completed the activity return to the next page and read on.

Worksheet 12 creating a session profile

SETTING UP WS_FTP

1 Start WS_FTP. As this is your first session, you will be asked to enter your e-mail address. Once you have done so, the Session Properties dialogue box (shown below) should appear.

Comment

WS_FTP comes with a list of FTP sites all ready to go, so you can just choose one of these from the Profile Name box and the program will try to connect you. If there's a particular site you want to visit that's not on the list, you'll have to set up a Session Profile for it first.

2 Point and click on the button labelled **New**.
3 In the Profile Name box, you can type any name to help you identify a site in the future. For our purpose type MenEpid.
4 In the Host Name/Address box, type the name of the computer you want to connect to. For our purpose type ftp.liv.ac.uk.
5 You can ignore the Host type box. WS_FTP will work it out for you.
6 As we are connecting to an anonymous FTP site, point and click the Anonymous box. This will place a checkmark in it. (If you were going to a private site, you would have needed to type your username in the User ID box.)
7 As we are entering an anonymous site, type guess in the Password box. (If you're visiting a private site, you will have typed your password. Also, if you don't want to enter your password each time you visit this site, you point and click on the **Save Pwd** to place a checkmark in it.)
8 Point and click the **Startup** tab. In the box labelled Initial Remote Host Directory, type the path to the directory you want to start in when connected. For our purpose type /pub/epidemic/ (don't forget that very first forward slash).
9 In the box marked Initial Local Directory, you can type the path to a directory on your own computer that you want any files to be downloaded. For our purpose type a:
Note: Every time you connect to this site drive a: will be selected.
10 Point and click on the **OK** button. WS_FTP will save these settings for future use and try to connect to the site when requested.

If you have completed the activity above, did you find any difference between the two methods of searching for a file on FTP sites?

The third method of reaching FTP sites is by using e-mail program. This is equally simple. All you need is to have a facility to send and receive e-mail.

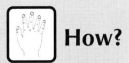

How?

using an e-mail program to get to ftp sites

If you have only e-mail access to the Internet you need not worry as you can still obtain the benefits of FTP. To access anonymous sites using your e-mail program, you simply log in with the username *anonymous* and give your e-mail address, or the word *guess*, as your password. Unfortunately, this versatility comes at a cost, can be tricky to manage, and first-time success is the exception rather than the rule (McKenzie, 1995).[16] (For further information on transferring files using e-mail, read McKenzie's book, Unit 19, pp. 143–7.)

7.2 using archie to find the health material you want

Note 'Archie' happens to be a famous cartoon character. The names of two other characters – 'Veronica' and 'Jughead' – from the same cartoon have been used to label two other search systems.

If you know what file you want and where to get it, then there is usually no big problem, as you would have already found out when you carried out Activities 7.1 and 7.2. However, the difficulty comes when you only have part of the information needed, then obtaining what you want may not be that easy at first. Take this scenario:

Suppose you have heard of a file or program that may help you with a particular health assignment you are researching, and luckily enough someone has told you the name and location of that file/program.

In the scenario above there is no problem: you simply type the URL into your browser's location box (like you did in Activities 7.1 and 7.2) and look for the file when the directory's contents are shown. But what if you only knew the location and not the name of the file? Then it is a bit like searching for a needle in a haystack. You could go to that location, enter the directory and view or download one of the Index files. This usually gives a short description of each file in that directory. With a bit of luck you might find the file you want.

However, if you knew the name of the file, and didn't know its location, the situation is much more promising but you may not necessarily want to spend hours searching computers. This is when you will appreciate what Archie can do for you. You can either use Archie on the web or a dedicated Archie program to connect to one of the **Archie servers**. Here are two of the best dedicated Archie programs:

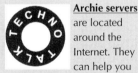

Archie servers are located around the Internet. They can help you find the exact location of the files you are looking for literally in seconds. These servers keep track of all the anonymous FTP public files on the Internet by searching the public directories of the FTP hosts on a regular basis and maintaining a list of all files.

- **WSArchie** – This program is the other half of the WS_FTP program mentioned earlier. For a free copy, visit this web site:

  http://www.mitredata.co.uk/wsarchie.html

- **fpArchie** – This program is even better because it does not need a separate FTP program. When it locates the file, it will download it for you. For a free copy of this program, visit this web site:

  http://www.euronet.nl/

Now try the activity below. It is designed to help you gain experience using Archie.

Activity 7.3   using archie to find a file

In Activity 7.1 you had all the essential information you needed, therefore you were able to locate the file: '*meningitis epidemic case study*'.

This time let's pretend that you only know the name of the file and nothing else. See if you can use Archie on the web or a dedicated Archie program to find it.

Do enlist someone on the Helpdesk to help you identify the *Archie program icon* on your college system. Activate it, then try to find the file mentioned above. Or if you are connected to the Internet at home, visit one of the web sites mentioned above and download *wsArchie* or *fpArchie*. Install the program on your computer system. Then try using it to find the file.

When you have completed the activity return to this page and read on.

How did you get on using Archie?

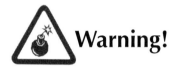 **Warning!** Although all Archie servers do much the same job, some find files that others don't. If a search ends in no results, choose a different server from the picklist of WSArchie's or fpArchie's drop-down menu. If you are unable to get to a particular Archie server because it is too busy, try again later.

7.3 gopherspace

Prior to the World Wide Web, the Gopher system was the friendly face of the Internet. It is an older Internet filing system that presents information as a series of menus. It consists of a number of computers around the world acting as Gopher servers (just as there are web servers, news servers, FTP servers and so on).

In Units 2 and 3, you were encouraged to explore the World Wide Web, and look at documents stored on web servers. In this section, you will be offered some information on connecting to Gopher servers and getting into 'Gopher-space' to search for documents.

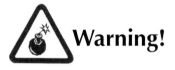 **Warning!** You are warned that nowadays you are unlikely to find many Gopher sites on the Internet – most have become web sites instead. The few remaining Gopher sites belong to universities, libraries, government departments, and other organizations that choose to continue to publish their information widely in simple form.

For any Gopher sites that you come across, you should find that your web browser should enable you to access them. Recognising Gopher sites is easy, as they have URLs that start with **gopher://**, for instance: Gopher://gopher.tc. umn.edu, which is the gopher of the University of Minnesota. Simply type the gopher URL in your browser's location box and provided it is properly configured you should be transported to your chosen site.

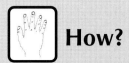

How?

how does a gopher work?

The Gopher server can be anywhere on the Internet. When you select an item on a menu, your service provider's computer sends a message to the remote Gopher telling it to send you that item. The process is similar to you requesting a catalogue from a company; you select an item from the catalogue, and then the company posts the chosen item to you. The difference is that with Gopher you do not get a bill at the end of the month.

Note Before attempting to access Gopher sites on your college system, you should check with the Computing department whether it has a Gopher client installed on the system.

If you are unable to access Gopher sites on your college system, and you are desperate to do so, you can always install a dedicated Gopher program like *WSGopher* on your home system. For more information, pay a visit to:

http://www.mstc.com

Connections between gophers are seamless, so you can move from one gopher to another without realizing it. You can retrieve text information from different parts of the world with equal ease.

7.4 telnet your way to nursing and medical information

Before we had Windows and the mouse, to use a computer you had to type commands from the keyboard. When the Internet became available for general use, people wanted to operate a computer at a distance; this gave birth to a service called Telnet. Telnet provides a facility that allows Internet users, like you, to log onto a remote computer, and give it instructions to perform, as if you were typing at the computer's own terminal. Although the Telnet service has been eclipsed by the flexibility of the World Wide Web, there are still many things you can use Telnet for. For example, you can read *e-mail* (Unit 5), access *Archie* (Unit 7), read *news* or *chat* (Unit 6) to other Internet users. You may also be able to log in and access your college/university computerized library catalogue from home.

The simplicity of Telnet makes it look boring. You get a command line, no graphics, and no sound (except for the occasional beep). However, the benefits are that it is simple to use and from the comfort of your home you can connect to other computers.

To use Telnet, you need a Telnet software installed on your PC, or your web browser set up to handle Telnet calls. As Telnet is unfortunately not a growing service, there are a limited number of Telnet programs around. Ewan (http://www.lysator.liu.se/~zander/ewan.html) is by far the best Telnet program. However, if you are using Windows 95/98/ME/2000/NT/XP, then you already have a good Telnet program incorporated and ready for use. In order to initiate a Telnet session, you need to know the address of the remote host computer. The syntax for using Telnet is:

telnet <address of remote host>

For example: **telnet libra.math.tau.ac.il**

This should initiate an interactive session with the libra server at the School of Exact Science at the Tel-Aviv University.

Many remote hosts require you to have an *account* to log in (i.e. you must have a user-id and a password). However, there are some remote hosts that do not require users to have an account. In these cases you can log in with the general user-id. (The password will usually be inserted automatically.) To gain experience of Telnet, Activity 7.5 offers a working example.

Activity 7.4 searching library catalogues from home

This activity will take you through the process of using your Windows95/98/ME/2000/NT/XP program to connect to an online library catalogue at the University of Miami, which maintains a database of AIDS health providers in southern Florida. The telnet address and password are as follows:

Telnet: **callcat.med.miami.edu**
Log in: **library**

When you reach the main menu, select 'P' (for 'AIDS providers') and you'll be able to search for doctors, hospitals and other providers that care for patients with AIDS. You can also search by speciality.

To help you carry out this activity, follow the step-by-step instructions listed in **Worksheet 13**.

When you have completed the activity return to this page and read on.

Worksheet 13 searching library catalogues from home

To connect to a remote computer library system you can use a dedicated Telnet program like Ewan or if you have Windows95/98/ME/2000/NT/XP installed on your home system, you can use the built in Telnet program.

CONNECTING TO A COMPUTERIZED LIBRARY SYSTEM (e.g. University of Miami, which maintains a database of AIDS health providers in southern Florida).

1 Start Windows.
2 Click on **Start** button. *A menu should pop-up.*
3 Click on the command **Run**. *A run dialogue box should appear.*

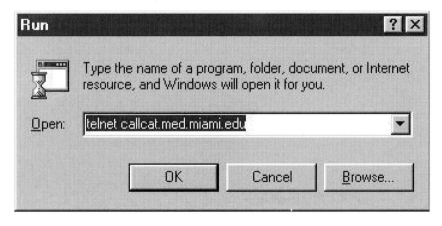

4 Type: **telnet** followed by the site's address.
(as we want to connect to the University of Miami AIDS database we type:)

telnet callcat.med.miami.edu

and click on the **OK** button.

5 If you are not already connected to the net, at this point you will be required to do so. *After a moment you should be connected to the host computer.*

6 When the library window appears, wait until you see a **'login'** prompt. (*Warning*: This may take a while.) Now, point and click next to it and then type the password which is: **library** then press the **ENTER** key.

7 Type the letter **'V'** in response to the question 'what kind of terminal are you using?' and then type **'Y'** to confirm.

8 At the main menu select **'P'** for AIDS providers, or **'L'** for library.

Using the appropriate Telnet address and password you may be able to Telnet into your own college/university library. However, as most colleges and universities are beginning to have a presence on the World Wide Web, an alternative way to access their library is to access their homepage and then click on a link that says 'library'. This way, from the comfort of your home you will be able to connect to your college/university library computer system to:

- Search the library catalogue
- Reserve any items out on loan
- Check your own borrower record and renew items
- Place inter-library loans.

This will save you the hassle of paying a bus fare or driving to your institution to find out if it has the books you want for your assignments. However, don't expect to be able to actually read the books online – maybe one day! For example, if you are a student at Canterbury Christ Church University College, you can use your home computer to access their library catalogue by doing the following:

1 Activate Windows.

2 Click on your browser's icon to get on the net.

3 In the **Address/Location** box type: http://www.cant.ac.uk

4 Click on the link that says **library**. *A new page should appear.*

5 Click on the option **library catalogue**. *A page similar to the screen shot below should appear.*

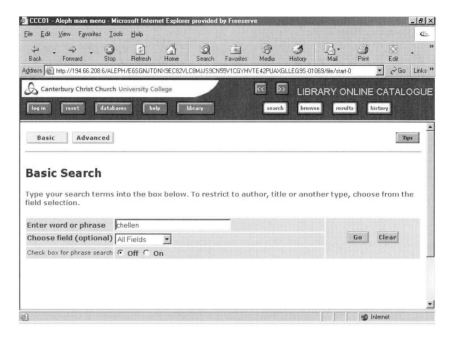

6 Type a word or phrase in the box provided (e.g. the name of an author) and then click the **GO** button.

Virtually all university libraries in the UK have a computerized catalogue, and the vast majority of these are accessible via the Internet. The same is also true for foreign universities. You can find a listing of UK and US libraries at:

http://library.usask.ca/hytelnet/

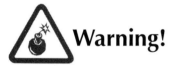

Public libraries are slower in connecting to the Internet. The British Library has its own online service, but in order to use the catalogue you will need to register. This will cost you a yearly fee. For more details go to the following web site:

http://portico.bl.uk/

summary and conclusion

Besides e-mail and WWW, there are additional tools such as *FTP*, *Archie*, *Gopher* and *Telnet* to help you get the best out of the Internet. For example, FTPs can be immensely helpful with your research project. You will also find that when you are in need of help finding the location of some pieces of information, Archie can do wonders for you. Finally with the right hardware and software at home you can Telnet your way into your institute's library in the comfort of your home.

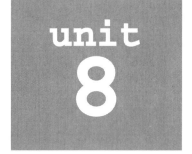

unit
8

publishing on the world wide web

I found it personally rewarding to design my first homepage, and then to upload it successfully to my Internet Service Provider. But the real satisfaction came when I was able to visit the site and view my efforts.

E. Newall (1999)[17]

Senior Lecturer Nursing Studies, Canterbury Christ Church University College,
Faculty of Health, Canterbury
http://www.enewall.free-online.co.uk

Now that you have learnt about the most essential services on the net and how to use them, they remain the creation of others. Having your own homepage is one of the best ways of publishing your ideas and creations to the world. You will find many service providers are keen and ready to enable you to create and maintain a homepage as part of your basic account. The mechanics of creating a web page are amazingly simple. Almost every software package you use can create HTML pages or images optimized for the web. But building a good web page is a little harder. The design need to be good, the pages need to be clear, relevant and compelling. It must be easy to find out what's on the site. Pleasing colour and good pictures can make a huge impact. In this unit, following an explanation of the most important component parts of a web page, you should be able to create a simple web page of your own. Included in this unit is a host of practical pointers that will help you get the most from you web site.

checklist

Below is a checklist of what you can expect to find out in this unit. Read through the statements then tick (✓) the items about which you would like to know more.

I would like to find out more about:

Please now read through the topics you have ticked.

HTML (HyperText Markup Language) is the language used to create web pages. The markup language is a set of codes or signs added to plain text to indicate how it should be presented to the reader, taking into consideration bold, italic or underlined text, typefaces to be used, beginning and ending of paragraphs, etcetera, etcetera, etcetera.

How?

how does html work?

Suppose you were using a word processor – like Word for Windows – to type a document, and you wanted a particular text in a sentence to appear in bold. To get the bold effect you simply highlight the desired text and click on the bold icon. You do not have to worry about the codes that make the word appear in bold. The word processor takes care of this for you and hides them from your view.

However, when you prepare a document to be displayed as a web page, and you wanted a particular text to appear in bold, you will need to type the appropriate code along with the text like this:

<B>**This is bold**</B> and this is plain

When the browser displays the web page containing that text, it uses the codes to show the bold feature like this:

This is bold and this is plain

Likewise, it uses other codes that you insert to show other features.

Tags are the HTML codes added to plain text in a document. This transforms it into a web page with full formatting and links to other files and pages.

These codes are known as **tags** and they consist of ordinary text placed between the less-than and greater-than signs. In the example above, the first tag, <B>, means 'turn on bold type'. Halfway through the sentence a second tag, </B>, is used meaning 'turn off bold type'. Notice that to turn off bold, the same tag is used again, but with a forward-slash inserted immediately after the less-than sign. There are several other codes, a few of which you need to be familiar with. Those codes are so logical that you should have no trouble remembering them. See Table 8.1 for a selected list.

To create a web page you need two of the following tools:

- A homepage wizard, or
- A web page editor like Internet Assistant for Word for Windows, or
- A text editor like Windows NotePad, or
- Any word processor which can store text in ASCII format,
- Plus a web browser to test out your pages and to get you on to the Internet.

Table 8.1
Formatting tags
and their functions

	A tag is distinguished from the rest of the text by being surrounded by < >.	
<HTML>	Use the tag on the left to indicate the beginning of a file, and use the one on the right to indicate the end of the file.	</HTML>
<HEAD>	Use the left and right tags to indicate the beginning and ending of a heading section.	</HEAD>
<TITLE>	Use the left and right tags to surround the title of the page.	</TITLE>
<BODY>	Use the left tag at the start of your content of the page and use the right tag to indicate the end of the content.	</BODY>
<B>	Use the left and right tags to turn on and off bold.	</B>
<I>	Use the left and right tags to turn on and off italic.	</I>
<U>	Use the left and right tags to turn on and off underlining.	</U>
<Hn>	There are six heading tags <H1> </H1> to <H6> </H6>. The text enclosed between the heading tags appears in that style. <H1> is the most prominent heading style. Use the left and right tags to surround a level *n* heading, where *n* stands for a number.	</Hn>
<FONT size=number>	Use this tag to state the size of the font. Number=1–7.	</font>
 	Use the tag on the left to indicate a line break. It does not need a closing tag.	
<P>	Use the left and right tags to split text into paragraphs.	</P>
<HR>	Use the tag on the left to draw a horizontal line across the page. This tag also causes a line break.	
<A HREF='linkname'>	Use the left tag to link your page to another web site. Replace the *linkname* by the URL of the web site you want to link to and replace the *texttolink* by a keyword or keyphrase.	</A>
<img src='URL'>	Use this tag to display an image.	
<Centre>	Use the left and right to put text in the centre of a line.	</centre>

Now, if you are ready to have a go at creating a simple web page then carry out Activity 8.1.

- Using Windows Notepad create a template and then use it to create a web page. For help on doing this, please follow the instructions in **Worksheet 14**.

When you have completed the activity read on.

Worksheet 14 creating a simple web page

CREATING A TEMPLATE

Comment

None of these tags do anything exciting by themselves but are very important in the construction of the web page. Your document has to be placed between the <HTML> and the </HTML> tags.

There are two chunks: the head (the section between <HEAD> and </HEAD> and the body (between <BODY> and </BODY>).

The head will contain the title inserted between the <TITLE> and </TITLE> tags and the body will contain the text you want to appear on your web page, and this will be typed between the <BODY> and </BODY> tags.

The body will also contain tags you need to display images, set colours, hyperlinks to other pages and sites and other things you want on your page.

1 Start **Notepad,** and then insert a <u>formatted</u> disk in drive A.
2 Type the text below:

```
<HTML>
<HEAD>
<TITLE>Untitled</TITLE>
</HEAD>

<BODY>
</BODY>
</HTML>
```

3 (For the purpose of this exercise) save this file to a **floppy disk** as **myweb1.htm**.

USING THE TEMPLATE TO CREATE A WEB PAGE

1 Replace the word Untitled with a suitable title for the document, for example **My homepage**.
2 Now, add some text to the page. You can copy what I have done below or replace it with your own entries.

```
<HTML>
<HEAD>
<TITLE>My homepage</TITLE>
</HEAD>

<BODY>
<H1>Welcome! </H1>
This is my first attempt at creating a web page.
<P> I hope you like it. </P>
</BODY>
</HTML>
```

Note

There are certain basic tags that will appear in almost every HTML document. We can start by making a 'template file' that we can use every time we want to create a new page. I will assume that you are using the Notepad program available in Windows.

3 When you've completed the above, ensure you have a formatted floppy disk in drive A.
4 Save the file to the **floppy disk** as **myweb2.htm**.
5 Close down Wordpad.

Now that you have created your web page it is time to view your creation. To do this, carry out Activity 8.2.

Activity 8.2   steps for viewing a simple web page

- Now to view your creation you need to use your browser. For help on how to do this, follow the instructions listed in **Worksheet 15**.

When you have completed the activity read on.

Worksheet 15   displaying a simple web page

DISPLAYING YOUR CREATION

1 Ensure the floppy disk on which you saved the file **myweb2.htm** is in drive A.
2 Open your browser (you do not need to be *online*).
3 Choose the command **File** on the menubar. *A submenu should drop down.*
4 Choose the command **Open**. *An Open dialog box should appear, and the cursor should be flashing in a white rectangular box.*

Fig. 8.1

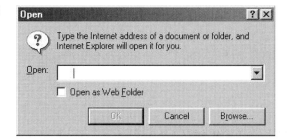

5 Type **a:\myweb2.htm** then click the **OK** button. *Your browser should display your creation, which should look like the screenshot below (Fig. 8.2).*

Fig. 8.2

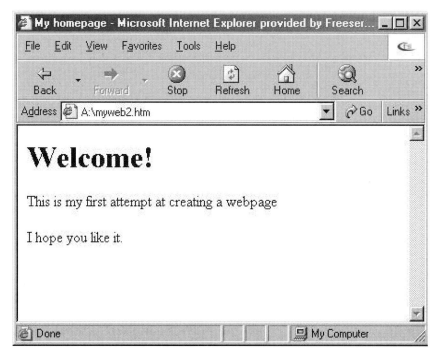

Although the web page you have created in the activities above is a simple one, it is just as easy to spice up that page by changing text size and font, adding links to other web pages, adding colour and background, and even pictures. The next activity will show you how to add a link to another site. Before we do that though, read the following subsections.

8.2.1.1 formatting text

For example, if you want to make your text **Bold**, *Italic* or <u>Underlined</u>, or all three, you simply surround the text with the appropriate tags like this:

I want to be <B>bold</B>. No, I prefer to be in <I>italic</I>. No, I want to be <U>underlined</U>. I really want to be <B><I><U>bold, italic and underlined</B></I></U>.

This is how your browser will display the above:

I want to be **bold**. No I prefer to be in *italic*. No I want to be <u>underlined</u>. I really want to be ***<u>bold, italic and underlined</u>***.

Since the tags <B> for bold, <I> for italic and <U> for underline have ongoing effects, you need to enter the closing tags </B>, </I>, and </U> to stop the effects.

8.2.1.2 heading tags

There are six heading tags that change the size of the text. <H1> is the most prominent heading style and <H6> is the least prominent. For example:

<H1> Welcome! </H1>

Welcome!

<H6> Welcome! </H6>

Welcome!

You can also use the *font* tag to change the font size. Sizes range from 1 to 7, with 1 being the smallest and 7 being the largest. For example:

<FONT SIZE=3> My homepage </FONT>

My homepage

8.2.1.3 inserting paragraphs and lines

The <BR> tag provides a line break without adding a line space. For example:

Welcome to . . .
 My homepage!

Welcome to . . .
My homepage!

The <P> tag also ends a line, but adds a line space. You should use this to split text into paragraphs. For example:

Welcome to . . . <P> My homepage!

Welcome to . . .

My homepage!

The <HR> tag divides the page into sections by drawing a horizontal line across the page. It also causes a line break. For example:

Mental Health Act:
<HR>
Section 2 – Admission for assessment
<HR>
Section 3 – Admission for treatment
<HR>
Section 4 – Emergency admission for assessment

Fig. 8.3

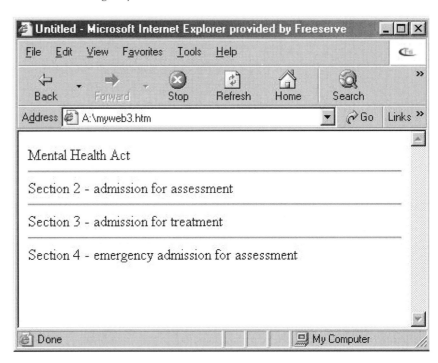

8.2.1.4 creating links to other sites

The hallmark of a good web site is that it should contain links to other web sites. To do this, you use link tags to add a *hyperlink* to other web pages. The link tag is:

<A HREF= '*link name*'> *texttolink* </A>

Here is an example:
Suppose you want to create a link from your web page (i.e. the one you created while doing Activity 8.1) to, say, the UK Department of Health web page. You can start a new paragraph and add the following:

<P> For more information visit the <A HREF='
http://www.open.gov.uk/doh/dhhome.htm'> *Dept. of Health* </A> site.

Figure 8.4 shows the result. The next activity will take you through the process of adding this link to your page. First, here is additional explanation about the link tag. In HTML, the link tags are referred to as 'anchors'. That's what the '**A**' after the first < sign means. An opening anchor usually begins with this tag:
<A HREF= '*link name*'>.

Instead of the *link name*, you type the URL of the page you want to link to, in between the quotation marks.

Immediately after the > sign, where it says ***texttolink***, you type in a keyword or keyphrase that you want visitors to your page to click on. Finally, you type in the closing anchor tag, </A>.

Now, have a go at Activity 8.2.

Activity 8.3 linking your web page to other web sites

It is assumed that you have completed *Activity* 8.1 and you saved your work using the filenames instructed.

Follow the instructions in **Worksheets 16** and **17**. They contain the steps for linking your web page to another web site.

When you have completed the activity return to this page and read on.

Worksheet 16 creating a link to another web site

ADDING A LINK ON YOUR WEB PAGE

1 Start Notepad.
2 Insert in **Drive A** the floppy disk containing the file **myweb2.htm**
3 Click the command **File** on the menubar. *A submenu should appear.*
4 Click on the command **Open**. *An Open dialog box should appear.*
5 In the Filename box type: **A:\myweb2.htm** then press ENTER. *The document you prepared earlier should now be loaded into Notepad.*
6 Now, modify the document so that it contains all the lines as shown below:

```
<HTML>
<HEAD>
<TITLE>My homepage </TITLE>
</HEAD>
<BODY>
<H1> Welcome! </H1>
This is my first attempt at creating a web page.
<P> I hope you like it </P>
<P> For more information visit the
<A HREF='http://www.open.gov.uk/doh/dhhome.htm'>
Dept. of Health </A> site.
</BODY>
</HTML>
```

7 For the purpose of this exercise save this file back to your **floppy disk** under a new file. I suggest: **myweb3.htm**.

1 Ensure the floppy disk on which you saved the file **myweb3.htm** is in drive A.
2 Open your browser (you do not need to be *online*).
3 Choose the command File on the menubar. *A submenu should drop-down.*
4 Choose the command **Open**. *An Open dialog box should appear, and the cursor should be flashing in a white rectangular box.*
5 Type the following: **a:\myweb3.htm** then press **ENTER**. *Your browser should display your new web page containing the link to the Department of Health, as shown in the screenshot below.*

Fig. 8.4 A web page containing a link to another web site

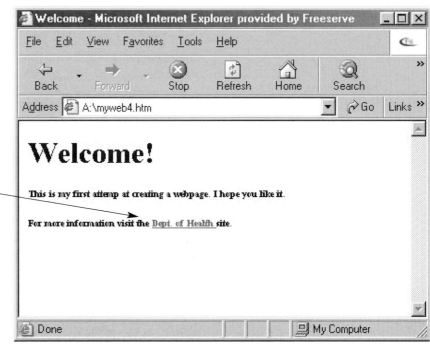

Comment
If you point and click on the keyphrase <u>Dept. of Health</u>, your browser should take you to that site.

Another type of anchor allows a visitor to your page to e-mail you from their web browsers. As the person clicks the link, it opens their e-mail message window, with your e-mail address already inserted, ready for them to send you a message. Suppose I wanted to create a link on my web page so that visitors can e-mail me, here is how I can do this:

<A HREF='mailto:s.s.chellen@cant.ac.uk'> Click here to send me an e-mail </A>

As you can see, I have replaced the URL with my e-mail address and I have also inserted the word **mailto**: immediately after that first quote sign. To do the same to your web page, simply use my example and replace my e-mail address with yours.

8.2.1.5 adding pictures

Another good way to spice up your web page is to add images. You will find lots of free high-quality graphics on the Internet. Here is a good site you can visit to hunt for free pictures:

- **Yahoo! Directory Web Graphics (Icons)**
  http://dir.yahoo.com/Arts/Design_Arts/Graphic_Design/Web_Page_Design_and_Layout/Graphics/Icons/

8.3 using html editors

I hope you enjoyed doing the activities set above. However, the process of generating web pages can be simplified by using an HTML editor. There are a few to choose from. These editors allow you to create HTML documents in a word-processing-like environment. They automatically produce complicated tags for graphics, frames, forms, lists, and tables. You can download most of the editors from the net. Here is a short list:

- **Navigator Gold** – Visit http://home.netscape.com/
- **FrontPage** – Visit http://www.microsoft.com/frontpage/
- **Pagemill** – Visit http://www.adobe.com/prodindex/pagemill/main.html

8.4 getting your web page on the net

Once you have created your web page you need to get in on the net. Transferring the files from your own computer onto the computer where your Internet account is located is called *uploading*. This is achieved by using an FTP utility, such as CuteFTP for Windows.

8.5 broadcasting your web page

Now that you have got you own web page you need to do some canvassing to get people to visit it. Here are a few ideas:

- Write to appropriate web sites and ask for a link
- Get on a Mailing list and announce it
- E-mail your friends and tell them about it
- Use free announcing services to promote your web page. Two of the best are:
  1 **Promote It** at http://www.iTools.com/promote-it/
  2 **UK Submit** at http://www.uksubmit.co.uk/

Whilst it is not hard to build a web page, building a 'good' one takes more effort. The last thing you want is to frustrate your visitors. Here are twenty practical pointers, adapted from Branscombe (2002),[18] to help you create a terrific web site.

1 **Be consistent** – Use the same background on every page and keep the home button in the same place. To make every page look different, you can vary the layout.

2 **Keep your visitors informed** – Visitors like to know where they are and where they are going next. Make sure the name or logo of your site is on every page. Mark all sections and label all links to other pages/sites clearly.

3 **Add FAQ** – If you are covering a subject that provokes questions, include a Frequently Asked Questions (FAQ) page. If you have got more than ten questions, organize them into sections.

4 **Eliminate guesswork** – Make it obvious how your site works. Do not force visitors to memorize inscrutable icons. Make it clear what is a link and where it goes. Only use the clearest images.

5 **Update** – Keep your site up-to-date and make it clear when it was last updated (and, if possible, when it is likely to be updated again).

6 **Simplicity is best** – Avoid going over the top when designing your page. It must be immediately obvious to any visitor how to use it, and how they can click tabs for more features.

7 **Start with essential info** – Most web users only read 200 words on screen. Only real enthusiasts look for all details. To cater for casual and enthusiast visitors, start with essential info and provide links for those who want to move on. Then add more details further down the page or on second page.

8 **Test it out** – Others will see things you have missed. Solicit comments from potential users (friends). Usually after five or so people you should see some patterns emerging.

9 **Go slow** – Just because you have a fast Internet connection does not mean that all your visitors are as lucky as you. Test your site on the slowest PC you can find, at 800 × 600 resolution and dial up with an ordinary 56k modem to see what your site really looks like.

10 **Web-friendly font** – Not every visitor will have extra fonts on their system, so pick a web-safe font for your web pages. This way all your visitors will enjoy the same appearance of your web pages. Remember that the point size of text looks different depending on which browser you use – Netscape shows text about one point smaller than Internet Explorer – and looks different again on a Mac. For very small text (6 or 7 point), use a style sheet to change the size for different browsers.

11 **Count it** – Adding a counter to your web site can be cool but remember that it will also slow down your site. If you really want to keep a log of the number of visitors to your web site, you should be able to find a free counter from: http://www.thecounter.com or you could pay for an invisible counter at http://counter.mycomputer.com.

12 **Pop-up windows** – Generally speaking visitors hate intrusive windows that pop-up on top of their browser. Avoid making windows open up without asking.

13 **Forms fill** – If you include a form, make it clear which fields are optional and which have to be filled in. If the form is incorrectly completed, indicate the areas that need correction before you can process it.

14 **Mind your colours** – (a) A lot of computers only use 256 colours. To make sure that the colour you choose is what your visitors see, keep within the basic 256 colours. (b) Do not use more than four or five colours (plus black and white) as this is likely to make your site look busy and overpowering. (c) Bright red or blue are hard to read – use less saturated colours for a more subtle look. (d) The standard hyperlink on a Web page is blue and under-lined. Don't change it without a good reason because you'll confuse inexperienced visitors. (e) Red gets attention and is good for error messages and warnings but too strong for background colour. Yellow is another attention grabber, but it tires your eyes quickly. Blue has a relaxing effect. (Note: colours have symbolic meanings that vary across the world: while we might think of white as the colour of purity, in Chinese culture it symbolizes death.)

15 **Use images with care** – When you insert a picture, fill in the ALT (Alternative text) tags, especially if it's a link. If visitors have images turned off, or if images don't load, they'll see the text. JPEG work best for images with a gradient of colours and continuous tones, like photos and paintings. JPEG take up less file space by losing some of the information in the picture. If you want to make it harder for people to copy images from your site, put watermarks and copyright notices on them.

16 **Keep your file sizes small** – Internet visitors tend to be quite impatient. To grab their attention you want your page to load fast. While the visitors are busy reading the text on one page, preload images for the next. Your web images should total no more than 30k maximum. If you have to use large images, make use of thumbnails and let the visitors decide which ones are worth viewing at full size.

17 **Keep it error-free** – It is sometimes hard to see mistakes in something you have written and read over and over. So make a print out and give it to someone else to read. Poor spelling and grammar is a sign of poor quality and this will put your visitors off.

18 **Qualify your icons** – When using graphics on navigation buttons, add text as well. Images on their own can be misleading. For example, a camera icon could mean a variety of things.

19 **Provide a search facility** – Help your visitors to find what you've got on your site. Try the following web site: http://www.freefind.com or http://www.fusionbot.com

20 **Make a map** – A site map showing all your pages should be clear and comprehensive. Many web editors have built-in site map tools, or you can use SiteXpert.

summary and conclusion

Now that you know how simple it is to create a web page, why not try creating your own and provide other health professionals/students in the world with the information you have been able to learn? It can be a really rewarding experience.

online help with your health studies and job search

The Internet is an almost infinite library that is constantly being updated. Users can often find the facts they seek in a few minutes, without leaving their desk, and at relatively low cost.

D. Couchman (1999)[19]

The Internet is a valuable tool for accessing all kinds of information. Nurses can use the Net for their studies and need to know how to reference Internet sources.

J. Howe (1998)[20]
Lecturer in Nursing, University of Wales College of Medicine,
School of Nursing Studies, Cardiff.

Universities and colleges were among the first sites to appear on the net. Online classes are slowly appearing. Some sites are giving information about examinations, tips for success, summaries of syllabuses, and so on. In this unit I seek to raise your awareness of a few interesting sites that could help you succeed in your course. Information will also be given on how to locate study tools, how to cite electronic sources and finally how to use the services on the net to find a job.

checklist

Below is a checklist of what you can expect to find out in this unit. Read through the statements then tick (✓) the items about which you would like to know more.

I would like to find out more about:

Please now read through the topics you have ticked.

Learning how to learn is a skill, and a skill well worth developing. If you have just returned to full or part-time education after a long break, you will find that there is material on the net to help you become a successful student. Take a visit to the Canterbury Christ Church University College homepage at <http://health.cant.ac.uk/students.htm>, from where you will be able to access a growing number of online tutorials and courseware. The page offers a comprehensive index of links to all such material.

Table 9.1

Online tutorials and courseware available at the Canterbury Christ Church University College web site

College Webmail
How to use college webmail and access your inbox

Exam Help
Look at past examination papers

IT Help
Access modules on a wide variety of IT skills

Web Sites
Hundreds of useful sites

Faculty Learning Resources
Support on using Faculty learning resources

Library Resources
Online catalogue and databases

University College Resources
Order books via college bookshop and online timetable

The section on 'Learning Information Skills with Technology' should prove particularly useful. It is designed to enable you to collect, analyse and present your findings. The development team who prepared that online course say 'this course is designed to support you acquiring a range of information skills that are fundamental to success with your course of study'. They also emphasise the importance of developing the skill to use NetScape effectively enough so that you can navigate around the pages in their online resource. At this web page

http://computing-services.cant.ac.uk/title

you will find several options at the top of the page. Some of them are listed in Table 9.2 below. You should find the sections *Learning and Teaching with Technology* and *Online IT tutorials* particularly useful.

Table 9.2

Materials available at the TiTLe web site

Information on TiTLe
A general statement on TiTLe and how to use it.

Learning and Teaching with Technology
Contains a guide which provides an introduction to academic staff on using technology in teaching and learning.

Online IT Tutorials
IT tutorials in pdf format for common college packages.

Training
Courses for staff and students.

ECDL
Provides details of the ECDL course.

As a student following an academic course in a college of higher education or university, you will have to write many essays. To complete these essays, you will be using, to some degree, your personal knowledge and, largely, information gathered from a variety of primary and secondary sources. It is important that you examine carefully the worth and arguments presented within those sources, particularly from those being published on the web.

9.2.1 the quality of information on the net

There is no quality control on the net. Anyone is free to put anything on the web and there is no requirement for anyone to prove to anyone what he or she is saying is indeed correct. Some of the material available may not be of a high academic or professional standard. It is left up to you to decide if what you find is reputable or not. A well-designed web site with colourful graphics and lengthy text are no assurance of quality. Table 9.3 offers three areas that you should look at and ask yourself a few questions:

Table 9.3
Evaluating web resources

Key areas	Questions	Comments
The author	**Who is the author?** Is (s)he a doctor, nurse, an academic, health organization, college/university, commercial company or interested individual? **What are the author's qualifications, experience and affiliation?** What qualifies the author to speak on this subject? Is (s)he highly regarded? Is the author affiliated to an organization? Are there possible biases as a result of his/her credentials and affiliation? **Why is the author providing the information?** Is it to support a college/ university course? Is it to sell a book, medical product or raise funds? Is it to provide unbiased information to patients?	It is said that 80% of the information on the net is rubbish. This implies there is 20% of useful information up for grab. Information about the author should help you evaluate the material. The 'About' pages usually explain who is providing the information and why. 'Disclaimers' and 'Copyright' statements indicate the limits on the material. The URLs give clues to the publisher or owner of the site. For example, **.ac.uk** indicates a UK academic site, **.edu** indicates a US academic site, **.co.uk** refers to a UK-based commercial site. Sections like 'History', 'Aims', 'Background' and 'About us' on a web page give you a clearer understanding of any organization and its functions.
The date	**When was the material published?** Is there a publication date? Is it recent or out of date? **How frequently is the web page updated?** Can you see a 'site updated' notice? Is the frequency of the update indicated? Do the links work? **How reliable is the site?** Are you confident that the site will be there tomorrow? Will you be able to track it down if the URL does change?	Theories and practice relating to health and medicine are in a constant state of change. Therefore, knowing the date of publication of any article, treatment guidelines, or patient information will help to ascertain the usefulness of the material. Almost anything that is more than ten years old should be treated with caution. The webmaster is a useful person to contact for queries, like when the site was last updated. Copyright statements may give a clue as to when material was first published.

Table 9.3 (*cont.*)

Key areas	Questions	Comments
The arguments and **The evidence**	**What points is the author attempting to make?** Is there clarity of thought? **What supportive evidence is offered?** Are statements supported by reliable evidence, such as research findings? Are findings from valid and respectable sources? **Where is the resource hosted?** Is it held on a commercial, educational or organizational server? Is it an individual's page on a university web site? Is it UK-based?	When writing your own academic essays, you will be borrowing ideas and facts from published material. Your assignment will be valued more if the points you make are backed up with references from reputable valid sources. A lot of health and medical web sites on the Internet are not UK-based. Using non-UK resources (especially US sites) may provide you with information that is not all that relevant. **Do not** use information from a site that cannot prove the validity of the information it offers.

9.3 referencing health material obtained from electronic sources

More and more data is now stored electronically in a variety of forms and in different types of location. Many of these locations are referred to as Internet sites.

The following are sources you are likely to encounter:

- Web sites
- Online databases
- FTP sites
- Personal e-mails
- Newsgroups
- Gopher sites
- Magnetic media like CD-ROMs and floppy disks.

When quoting, your sources may be in one or more of the above forms. Being able to reference your sources clearly is an important aspect of writing academic assignments. A little time spent in understanding what is expected of you will pay dividends.

9.3.1 what is meant by referencing?

In gathering information from print sources (such as books, journals, conference papers . . .) and from electronic sources (such as CD-ROMs, the web and so on), you will use the ideas, facts and opinions of others to support your arguments in your written assignments. On occasion you will also use the exact words that particularly support the topic you are considering in your essay. As you draw on these sources you will be expected to acknowledge the origins of the information or quotations you incorporate into your academic work. Presenting information obtained from the works of others as if it is your own is plagiarism – a habit you should avoid at all costs because it is one of the most serious academic 'crimes' you could commit in educational settings.

You will avoid plagiarism by crediting the author whose ideas and opinions you have borrowed. References relate to a list of works cited within the text and included at the end of your written work. Two important reasons for compiling that list are:

- It enables readers – and markers – of your work to trace (and check) the source material.
- It also demonstrates that you have not just given your own opinions but have also included other opinions to illustrate a point or offer support for an argument.

9.3.2 formats of references

A **reference list** can be defined as the bibliographical details of documents that support statements made in the main body of the essay/thesis.

A **bibliography** is a list of background reading carried out for the assignment but not cited as direct reference in the body of the essay. NB materials should be listed in alphabetical order, with full details as for direct references. Most institutions prefer that the bibliography list is headed 'Bibliography' and is kept separate from the 'Reference list'.

In preparing your written work, you should use the style of referencing specified by your institution. If you are not sure which one to use, check with your course tutor. The Harvard and the Vancouver styles continue to be the two most commonly used systems for referencing printed materials within books and periodicals. Here is a quick reminder of those two styles of referencing as they are applied to printed materials.

- **Harvard system:** This system is often referred to as the 'author/date' system (Dwyer, 1995),[20] and is used mainly in nursing and the social sciences (Bournemouth University Library, 1999).[21] When using this system, if the author's name occurs naturally in the sentence, references are cited in the main body of the text like this: Chellen (1995) wrote about the . . . ; otherwise like this: (Chellen, 1995) at the end of the sentence. This is then listed alphabetically by surname in a reference list at the end of the work. This reference list follows a general form as illustrated in Table 9.4.
- **Vancouver system:** This system is also referred to as the 'numerical system' (Dwyer, 1995). When using this system – which most academic/medical journals prefer – references are numbered consecutively in the text and are listed in numerical order at the end of the essay/paper. The reference list follows the general form as illustrated in Table 9.4.

Table 9.4
Citation systems
for books and periodicals

	Harvard style	Vancouver style
BOOKS	Author(s)/editor surname, initials. (Year of publication) Title of book, edition [if later than first]. Place/town of publication: Publisher's name.	(No.) Author/s, Initials, *Title*. (Edition). City: Publisher, Year: (Page numbers)
	Example: Chellen, S.S. & Chellen, P.D. (1995) *Word for Windows for the Caring Professions – A Beginner's Workbook.* London: Cassell plc.	**Example**: (1) Chellen, S.S. & Chellen, P.D. *Word for Windows for the Caring Professions – A Beginner's Workbook.* London: Cassell plc. 1995.
ARTICLES	Author(s) surname, initials (Year of publication) Article title. *Journal title.* Volume number (issue number) Date and month of issue: first and last pages.	(No.) Author/s. Title {Type of article}. *Journal*, Year, Month, Date; Volume (Issue): Page numbers.
	Example: Chellen, S.S. (1995) A Layman's Guide to IT, in *Occupational Health – a Journal for Healthworkers*, 47(10), 10 Oct: pp. 351–2 & 354–5.	**Example**: (2) Chellen, S.S. A Layman's Guide to IT, in *Occupational Health – a Journal for Healthworkers*, 1995. Oct 10; 47(10): 351–2 & 354–5.

 Note In the examples given, note:
1 The order
2 Where there are capital letters
3 What is in italics/underlined
4 Punctuation.

N.B. Notice that some words are underlined. Underlining is used if the assignment is hand written or typed on a conventional typewriter. Use italics if the assignment is wordprocessed.

For more information on Harvard style visit:

http://library.cant.ac.uk/citing-references.htm
[accessed 27 November 2002]

http://www.sghms.ac.uk/depts/is/library/int_res/electr.htm
[accessed 20 December 2002]

Information on electronic sources can be classified under two broad headings: 'Internet Sources' and 'Non-Internet Sources'. The first category includes material from electronic journals, individual works on web sites, personal e-mail, mailing lists, newsgroups, FTP sites, Gopher sites, and online databases. The second category includes material from electronic media like CD-ROMs and computer disks.

Unfortunately, as yet there is no agreed and fixed standard for referencing Internet publications, but it is slowly emerging. One particular problem is the temporary nature of much of the material made available on the Internet. This makes it hard for the scientific community to decide whether it can accept the validity of a non-permanent document as a legitimate reference source. Indeed, writers like McKenzie (1996, p. 55)[22] have rightly argued that only archived, retrievable versions may be regarded as valid. But, as electronic sources become an intrinsic part of your scholarly interaction, it is essential when referencing these sources that you do so with the same degree of care as for printed material.

To assist you, various writers have suggested ways of adapting the Harvard and Vancouver systems to apply them to electronic sources. Below is my adaptation of the two systems, offered as a guide only. You should also consult the course handbook in your institution. To allow your source to be checked and verified, you should cite the reference in the text in the same way as you would for printed materials, and then use the format indicated in Table 9.5 to list the references making sure to include all the information given in

Subsection 9.3.2.1 below.[23] When citing electronic references, accuracy is very important. A simple error like a full stop in the wrong place can make a reference listing useless. Below are seven keypoints worth bearing in mind.

7 keypoints to remember when listing references

1 Details of Internet sites or addresses should be recorded with *complete* accuracy.
2 All use of capital and lower case letters must be respected.
3 All punctuation must be recorded exactly as given.
4 No punctuation should be *added*. For example, do not put a full stop at the end of an address:

http://www.cant.ac.uk

not

http://www.cant.ac.uk**.**

5 All typographic symbols (#,@,!,~) should be incorporated accurately.
6 You should include a record of the date you visited the site.
7 Electronic documents may easily be updated at any time.

9.3.2.1 essential information required in reference citations

When citing references you need to include at least the following bibliographical details:

- Author
- Date
- Title
- Medium
- Location
- Commands.

> **Note** Inserting a date can be problematic as material on the net is dynamically updated. Furthermore, the 'dd/mm/yy' date convention is not followed by everybody; the suggestion is to use April 12 (as opposed to 12/04/97, which can be interpreted as December 4) (McKenzie, 1996, p. 55). Page numbers are not usually a feature of electronic documents, as pages will change depending on the viewing method.

Author: The name(s) of the person(s) or publishing body responsible for the document. This is usually the first element of a citation. If the author is not available, the title becomes the first element of the reference, and the work is alphabetized in the reference list by the first significant word in the title.

Date: The year, month and day when the electronic form of the publication was created or updated and/or accessed. This validates the existence of a cited file at a given time, and indirectly indicates the possible version of, say, a database when this becomes difficult to determine. The access date element is always the last element of a citation and enclosed in square brackets. This allows for later modification or removal of information.

Title: This is the main heading on the electronic document being cited or in the Titlebar, i.e. the blue strip at the top of the screen. If later than the first, this should include an edition or version number.

Medium:	This is the type of resource the information is stored on, e.g. online, CD-ROM, Laserdisk, Videodisk, Diskette, e-mail, WWW, etc. This is to show that the reference source is not a printed book or article. In situations where it is difficult to detect the medium, for example when using a database on a college computer network, then use the generic term 'electronic' to distinguish the cited electronic references from print ones.	
Location:	Wherever the user has to go to in order to find the document in question, e.g. http, ftp address, etc. The golden rule here is accuracy. Be extra careful with spelling and punctuation.	
Commands:	Any other instructions needed to locate the document (if relevant).	

9.3.3 referencing internet sources

Table 9.5a
World Wide Web and electronic journals

	Harvard style	Vancouver style
	Author(s), Initials. (Date created/ updated). Document Title. [Medium]. Location. [Date, Month, Year accessed]	(No.) Author(s), Initials. Document Title. [Medium]. Year. Location. [Date, Month, Year accessed]
Example 1	ENB Report On Practice Placement Review Visits – Learning Disability Nursing MAY 1997–APRIL 1998. [WWW]. Available from: <http://www.enb.org.uk/ldplace.htm> [Accessed: 27 November, 1998]	(1) ENB Report On Practice Placement Review Visits – Learning Disability Nursing MAY 1997–APRIL 1998. [WWW]. Available from: <http://www.enb.org.uk/ldplace.htm> [Accessed: 12 January,1999]
Example 2	Allen, M. (no date). SPSS for Windows Version 7 – A review. In *On-line Journal of Nursing Informatics* 1(1). [WWW]. Available from: <http://cac.psu.edu/~dxm12/spss. html> [Accessed: 15 January, 1999]	(1) Allen, M. SPSS for Windows Version 7 – *A review in On-line Journal of Nursing Informatics* 1(1). [WWW]. Available from: <http://cac.psu.edu/~dxm12/spss. html> [Accessed: 15 January, 1998]
Comments	• Often the author's name, or a link to the author's homepage, can be found at the bottom of the web page. In some cases, the author may be the organization responsible for the site. • Many WWW pages now include the date when it was last updated, which is equivalent to the publication date. If not, make sure you include the date you accessed the page. • The title of a web page will normally be the main heading on the page, or in the Titlebar, i.e. the blue strip at the top of the screen. • When including URL it is best to use angle brackets (< >) around the URL to set it off. Without such delimiters, inexperienced readers may misinterpret following punctuation as part of the URL (even though URLs shouldn't end in full stops, commas, or semicolons). Also only move to a new line following a forward slash(/). • Use a name, not a number, for the host part of the URL. For example: http://www.eeicom.com/eye/, not <http://204.7.7.4/eye/> • Remember URLs are case sensitive, i.e. they recognize the difference between upper and lower case. Make sure they are given accurately. • Some web pages are part of a larger set of documents, such as an electronic journal or book; for them it may be appropriate to include the title of the larger publication.	

Table 9.5b	Harvard style	Vancouver style
Online databases	Author(s), Initials. (Date created/updated). Document Title. [Medium]. Location. [Accessed: Date, Month, Year]	(No.) Author(s), Initials. Document Title. [Medium]. Year/Month/Date. Location. [Accessed: Date, Month, Year]
Example 1	Cort. E. (no date) Nurses' attitudes to sexuality in caring for cancer patients. In *Nursing Times*, 21 Oct. 1998, 94(42): pp. 54–6. [Online ENB Healthcare Database]. Available from: <http://www.enb.org.uk/cgi-bin/hcdsearch>. In Search box type: CANCER PATIENTS. [Accessed: 2 February 1999]	(1) Cort. E. Nurses' attitudes to sexuality in caring for cancer patients. In *Nursing Times*, 21 Oct. 1998, 94(42): pp. 54–6. [Online ENB Healthcare Database]. Available from: <http://www.enb.org.uk/cgi-bin/hcd> In Search box type: CANCER PATIENTS. [Accessed: 2 February 1999]
Example 2	Chellen, S.S. (1995) A Layman's Guide to IT. In *Occupational Health: A Journal for Occupational Health Nurses* 47(10): pp. 351–2, 354–5. [Online Database: CINAHL]. Available from Electronic Services – BIOMED: <http://biomed.niss.ac.uk> Select Author then type: Chellen. [Accessed: 5 February 1999]	(2) Chellen, S.S. A Layman's Guide to IT. In *Occupational Health: A Journal for Occupational Health Nurses* 47(10): pp. 351–2, 354–5. 1995. [Online Database: CINAHL]. Available from Electronic Services – BIOMED: <http://biomed.niss.ac.uk> Select Author then type: Chellen. [Accessed: 5 February 1999]
Comments	• *To facilitate location of the article, it is extremely important to include the keyword or keyphrase you used to access the article in the database.*	

Table 9.5c	Harvard style	Vancouver style
FTP sites	Author(s), Initials. (Date created/updated). Title of document or file. Edition/Version [Medium]. Location. [Accessed: Date, Month, Year]	(No.) Author(s), Initials. Title of document or file. Edition/Version. [Medium]. Year. Location. Accessed: Date, Month, Year]
Example	RANKIN, B (1997, Jan 27). Accessing the Internet by e-mail, (6th ed.). [FTP]. Available from: <ftp://ftp.mailbase.ac.uk/pub/lists/lis-iis/files/e-access-inet.txt>	(1) RANKIN, B Accessing the Internet by e-mail, (6th ed.). [FTP]. Available from: <ftp://ftp.mailbase.ac.uk/pub/lists/lis-iis/files/e-access-inet.txt>
Comments	• *When including the URL use angle brackets (< >) around the URL to set it off and only move to a new line following a forward slash (/).* • *Use a name, not a number, for the host part of the URL.*	

Table 9.5d

Gopher sites	Harvard style	Vancouver style
Gopher	Author(s), Initials (Date created/ updated). Document Title. Version/ Format. [Medium]. Location. [Accessed: Date, Month, Year]	(No.) Author(s), Initials. Document Title. [Medium]. Year. Location. [Accessed: Date, Month, Year]
Example	MIT Center for Space Research (1997, Jan. 20) Space Shuttle News. [Gopher]. Available from: Gopher://gopher.umds.ac.uk:70/00 technical/space-shuttle-news	(1) MIT Center for Space Research Space Shuttle News. [Gopher]. 1997. Available from: <Gopher://gopher.umds.ac.uk:70/00/ technical/space-shuttle-news>
Comments	*Refer to Table 9.5c.*	

Table 9.5e

Personal e-mail messages (archived works)

	Harvard style	Vancouver style
	Author(s), Initials (date posted). Subject line from posting. [Medium]. Location. [Accessed: Date, Month, Year]	(No.) Author(s), Initials. Subject line from posting. [Medium]. Date Posted. Location. [Accessed: Date, Month, Year]
Example	RIUS-RIU, M (1998, May 22) Copyright on the Internet [Personal e-mail to Chellen. SS]. Available from: <ssc1@cant.ac.uk>] [Accessed: 23 May 1998]	(1) RIUS-RIU, M. Copyright on the Internet [Personal e-mail to Chellen. S.S.]. 22 May 1998. Available from: <ssc1@cant.ac.uk> [Accessed: 23 May 1998]

Comments

- *When including an Address use angle brackets (< >) around the address to set it off.*
- *If your source is controversial or temporary then keep a hard copy, just in case you are requested to produce it. Better still attach a hard copy to your essay, thesis, etc.*
- *Personal e-mail should be treated in a similar manner to other non-electronic forms of personal communication. It is essential to request permission from the author before quoting an e-mail message in essays, especially if you are including the author's e-mail address, otherwise, as Steve Gilligan (see earlier, p. 124) points out, you may break both Copyright and Data Protection regulations.*

Table 9.5f

E-mail messages from usenet newsgroups

	Harvard style	Vancouver style
	Author(s), Initials (date posted). Subject line from posting in newsgroups. [Medium]. Newsgroup name.	(No.) Author(s), Initials. Subject line from posting in newsgroups. Date posted. [Medium]. Newsgroup name.
Example	Strong, A. (1998, December 26) Clinical Assistant: A new nursing role? [Usenet]. Available from: <uk.sci.med.nursing>	(1) STRONG, A. Clinical Assistant: A new nursing role? 26 December1998. [Usenet]. Available from: <uk.sci.med.nursing>

Comments

- *Use posting date, to allow tracing of message through archives.*
- *The title is the subject line/header.*

Table 9.5g	Harvard style	Vancouver style
E-mail messages from mailing lists	Author(s), Initials (date posted). Subject line from posting on listname. [Medium]. Server host address.	(No.) Author(s), Initials. Document Title. Date posted. [Medium]. Server host address.
Example	MACLEOD, R. (1996, January 19). Internet resources Newsletter – latest issue on LIS-LINK. [Mailing Lists]. Available from: <mailbase@mailbase.ac.uk>	(1) MACLEOD, R. Internet resources Newsletter – latest issue on LIS-LINK. 19 Jan. 1996. [Mailing Lists]. Available from: <mailbase@mailbase.ac.uk>
Comments	• *The title is the subject line.* • *By using posting date, it allows tracing of the message through archives. However, such messages although archived are often kept for a short time. Consequently, some institutions may not consider this source as suitable for referencing.*	

9.3.4 referencing non-internet sources

Table 9.5h	Harvard style	Vancouver style
Computer disks	Author(s), Initials. (Date created/ updated). Document Title. [Medium]. Version. Town. Publisher.	(No.) Author(s), Initials. Document Title. Version. Date created/updated. [Medium]. Town. Publisher.
Example	Education and Training Programme in IM & T for Clinicians (1996, Sept.) Champion Database. Version 3.2. [Disk]. Bristol: Blackwell Idealist.	(1) Education and Training Programme in IM & T for Clinicians Champion Database. Version 3.2. September 1996. [Disk]. Bristol: Blackwell Idealist.

Table 9.5i	Harvard style	Vancouver style
CD-ROM databases	Author(s), Initials. (Date created/ updated). Document Title. Version. [Medium]. Town. Publisher.	(No.) Author(s), Initials. Document Title. Version. Date created/updated. [Medium]. Town. Publisher.
Example	Caredata CD: the social and community care database. [CD-ROM]. 1997, April. London: National Institute for Social Work.	(1) Caredata CD: the social and community care database. [CD-ROM]. April 1997. London: National Institute for Social Work.

Table 9.5j CD-ROM texts	Harvard style	Vancouver style
	Author(s), Initials. (Date created/ updated). Document Title. Version. [Medium]. Town. Publisher.	(No.) Author(s), Initials. Document Title. Version. Date created/updated. [Medium]. Town. Publisher.
Example 1	Using Technology to find Clinical Information. [CD-ROM]. 1998, April. Bristol: Enabling People Team NHS Executive – South & West. Tel 0117 984 1904.	(1) NHS Executive Using Technology to find Clinical Information. [CD-ROM]. April, 1998. Bristol: Enabling People Team NHS Executive – South & West. Tel 0117 984 1904.
Example 2	Using IM & T in Clinical Practice. [CD-ROM]. 1998, April. Bristol: Enabling People Team NHS Executive – South & West. Tel 0117 984 1904.	(2) Using IM & T in Clinical Practice. [CD-ROM]. April,1998. Bristol: Enabling People Team NHS Executive – South & West. Tel 0117 984 1904.
Example 3	Mathers, L.H., Chase, R.A., & Dev, P.A. (1996, Oct.). Clinical Anatomy Interactive Lesson. [CD-ROM]. St Louis: Mosby.	(3) Mathers, L.H., Chase, R.A., & Dev, P.A. Clinical Anatomy Interactive Lesson. Oct., 1996. [CD-ROM]. St Louis: Mosby.
Comments	*In examples 1 and 2 above, the title is the first element of the reference. In the reference list for the Harvard style, the work is alphabetized using the first significant word in the title.*	

9.4 finding a health or health-related job online

After all your hard work and successful completion of your course, you quite rightly would like to be rewarded with a suitable job. This can be a very trying time. Once again you will find the net coming to your rescue.

- Take a visit to 'The PeopleBank' the following at: http://www.peoplebank. com where you will find thousands of vacancies in the UK.

Fig. 9.1 The PeopleBank homepage
Here as a jobseeker you won't have to pay anything. Simply fill in the online registration form, and submit your CV or browse through the database of job vacancies.

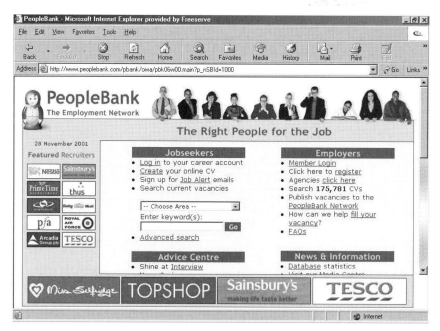

- **Or** visit **TotalJobs** at:

  http://www.totaljobs.com/jobseekers/totaljobs.asp

Fig. 9.2a Looking for a job on the totaljobs web site

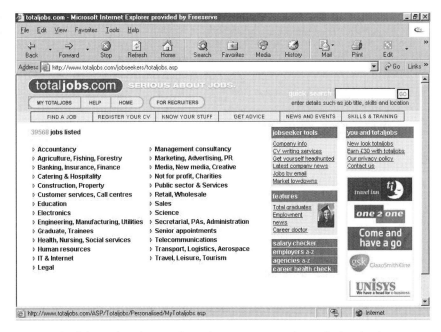

Here to find the right job, simply pick a category and search the database.

Step 1

1 Type the URL given above in the **Address/Location** box, and then press the **Enter** key. *A screen similar to the one above should appear.*

2 Point and click on the category labelled **Health, Nursing, Social services**. *You will be taken to the next screen shown below.*

Fig 9.2b

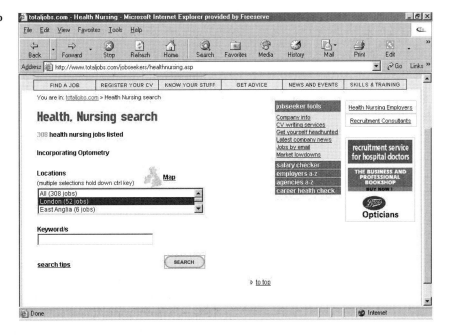

Step 2

1 Select a location, such as London. *Your chosen location will be highlighted as shown in the screenshot.*

2 Point and click on the **Search** button. *You will be taken to the next screen as shown below.*

Fig. 9.2c

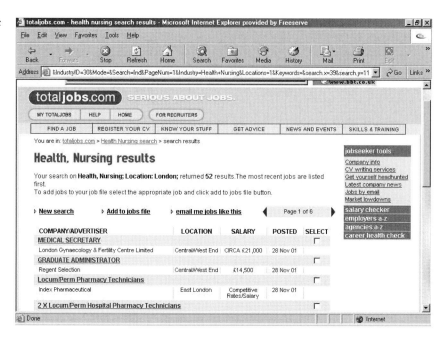

Step 3

• Now simply follow the onscreen instructions.

The site also features an easy-to-use salary checker, a huge database of company profiles, a career doctor, and a free career health check questionnaire.

• Other UK's best job hunting sites are:
  Fish4jobs at http://fish4.co.uk/jobs – This site was developed by a consortium of five major media groups – together representing around 80 per cent of the UK's local newspapers. Fish4jobs lists more than 30,000 jobs per day, most of which are sourced from the papers themselves. You will find a nice variety of career advice, including links to online courses and psychometric tests. You can save your search results in a personal folder and have new vacancies e-mailed to you.
  Monster.co.uk at http://www.monster.co.uk – This site lists 25,000 British jobs. It is part of a large international network of sites and features a number of added facilities, including free e-mail alerts and an online CV-building service. If you have been wrongly dismissed, you will find a section covering the law surrounding wrongful dismissal. If you are seeking a job abroad, then you will be impressed with the global listings containing over one million vacancies overseas.
  Workthing.com at http://www.workthing.com – This is a great site owned by the Guardian Media Group. It contains a salary checker, CV assessment quiz and job e-mail delivery. After you have registered, you can use the matrix to save search criteria and see an at-a-glance breakdown of jobs.

- Subscribe to newsgroups, and filter the newsgroup list. Useful ones are alt.jobs; alt.jobs.overseas; uk.jobs; sci.med.jobs.

- If you subscribe to a mailing list, you might be pleasantly surprised to see job vacancies being automatically delivered to your mailbox.

You can also scan professional journals online. Go to http://yahoo.co.uk/ and type the keyphrase **british journal** in the search box and then press the Enter on the keyboard.

9.4.1 getting started

Start by writing several CVs and tailor them to every job you apply for. Remember that your CV has but one purpose: to get you an interview. Sometimes you can submit your CV directly to potential employers via the web or e-mail, but some companies/institutions still prefer to receive job applications in writing. When submitting a CV online, supply it as both a formatted *Word* document and as *plain* (ASCII) text – just to be certain that it's readable. When printing your CV, print on one side only and ensure it is no longer than two A4 sides. This way it will be easier to photocopy and fax. If you are using your employer's computer and you do not wish him/her to know that you're job hunting, use a *web-based* e-mail like Hotmail for your correspondence (see Section 5.8). When applying by e-mail, do not expect an immediate reply or acknowledgement. Some will respond by e-mail, snail-mail or will phone after a few days.

summary and conclusion

Online tutorials can provide a valuable way of developing your skills in learning. By all means use the health information on the net to help in your assignments, but do take care with this, as the information may not be reliable. Be extra careful when referencing sources from the net. The Internet provides yet another way of job hunting.

twelve big questions and answers

Question 1 what is a pdf document?

Answer: Documents can be saved to disks in a variety of formats. When accessing online journals, such as *Nursing Standard Online*, you will find that some documents have been prepared in a special format called Adobe PDF, which stands for 'Portable Document Format'. To view, navigate, and print such documents, you need a special program called Acrobat Reader. You should find this program on the desktop of your college computer network. Adobe Acrobat Reader is usually available free of charge. Your college computing department should be able to give you a copy to use on your home system. If not, you can always visit the Adobe web site http://www.adobe.com/products/acrobat/readstep.html and download a free copy.

   When you come across a PDF document, you will first have to save it to disk using a unique filename. Then to read it, do the following:

- Activate the Acrobat Reader program
- Choose **File** from the menubar
- Choose the command **Open**
- In the **Open File** dialogue box, highlight the filename, and click on the command **Open**. *The article you saved should open into the Acrobat Viewer window.*

> **Note** Normally a PDF document has the extension **.pdf**. In Windows (or on the Macintosh) you can also open a PDF document by double-clicking the file icon. If double-clicking a file on the Macintosh platform does not open the file in your Acrobat Viewer, use **File | Open** to open the file, then close the file, and try again.

Question 2 what are cookies?

Answer: Cookies are small text files that are stored on your computer's hard disk when you visit certain web sites. They serve a variety of purposes for the author of a web site and can be of some benefit to those who visit the site. For example, when you have visited a web site and accepted a Cookie, a unique code that identifies you is saved to your hard disk. An advantage of having accepted a Cookie is that when you revisit the site, you may not be required to go through the process of supplying your name and password. You may even be allowed to access restricted areas of a site. Web creators (particularly those who rely on advertisements for their income) often use Cookies to keep a log of the paths you follow through the site and the pages you decided to visit. This helps them to know a bit more about your interests, and enables them to target you with the kind of adverts most likely to capture your attention. When you visit certain web sites for the first time, a dialogue box will appear offering you a Cookie. You have the choice of accepting or rejecting the offer by clicking on the appropriate option. Cookies are quite safe. Contrary to popular belief, they can't be used to spy on you, i.e. read any other data from your hard disk or find out what software you have installed.

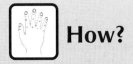
how does cookie work?

Cookies work like this: When you are surfing the web pages and follow a link to re-visit a web site, your browser sends the Cookie containing the URL of the site as you click the hyperlink. This immediately informs the site that you have been there before. You may receive a nice personalized welcome, such as 'Hello Syd, this is your third visit'.

Although Cookies are quite harmless, you may object to the fact that others are attempting to use your hard disk to store those small text files. Fortunately, you can set your browser to warn you when a site is attempting to store a Cookie on your hard disk. A dialogue box may appear containing the following message:

> In order to provide a more personalized browsing experience, will you allow this Web site to put information on your computer?
>
> If you click Yes, the web site will save a file on your computer. If you click No, the current web page may not display correctly.
>
> **YES   NO   More Info**

Sadly, when you decide to reject a Cookie you may find that some sites will not let you in. A smarter way of dealing with Cookies is to accept them and then delete them when you have finished surfing.

To locate and view Cookies

- Open your Windows directory folder, and then. . .
- Open the Cookies directory folder.
- Point and double-click on a Cookie header to open its contents into a window for reading.

To delete a Cookie

- Point to the Cookie header and click the RIGHT mouse button to open the submenu.
- Click on the **Delete** command on the submenu to get off that Cookie.

Question 3   what are computer viruses and are they harmful?

Answer: There will be occasions when you will be using your college computer network to download information from the net to take home to use on your computer system. Similarly there may be times when you may start preparing your assignment on your home system and then decide to finish it off on the college computer network or vice versa. The risk of exporting or importing a virus is real. So what is a computer virus? It is a category of software which infects other software programs and data files, and which replicates itself. A virus can spread via disks and the main problem is usually its side effects. Viruses have been known to transmit themselves over an entire network. There are over 200

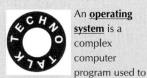

An **operating system** is a complex computer program used to control, assist or supervise all other programs that run on a computer system.

viruses at large and the number is steadily growing. Among these, 95% simply replicate themselves, cause your keyboard to beep every time you hit a key on your keyboard on a particular day of the month, or display a message on your computer screen. However, a minute few can be problematic. The most serious type is the one that infects an **Operating System** as this governs the whole running of a computer system. Fortunately, there are vaccine programs that can deal with viruses. Although virus infections can be regarded as just another PC problem, the more preventive measures you can take against viruses entering a system the better, since getting rid of a virus can take time, and time is money. Table Q1 outlines ways of minimizing the risk. For additional information read Section 5.9 and pay a visit to Dr Solomon's web site:

http://drsolomon.com

Table Q1
How to protect your computer system against viruses

Software	Use only software that comes from reputable sources. Avoid using pirated versions of software.
Compartmentalization	Keep program files and data files in separate directories or better still on separate disks.
Vaccine	Inoculate your computer against known viruses.
Virus guard	Install a virus guard on your computer.
Backups	Maintain regular backups of all your files.
Screening	Ensure that any disk you receive or bring home with data is virus-free by checking it using the latest version of a virus-checking program like Dr Solomon.
Performance	You should investigate and rectify any flaws in a widely used program as soon as they come to light.
Access control	Prevent unauthorized access to your data files or programs by using access controls such as passwords.

Question 4   what are plug-ins?

Answer: Web pages are getting smarter and smarter. Web site creators are increasingly making imaginative use of multimedia facilities. However, your browser may not be able to support these novelties. Plug-ins are software programs that extend the capabilities of your web browser in a certain way, such as allowing you to hear live audio broadcasts or view video movies. A plug-in is installed on your hard disk using the instructions that come with the plug-in. After installation your NetScape browser uses the plug-in's capabilities like other built-in NetScape features. There are literally hundreds of plug-ins out there to enable you to access different types of multimedia file. For example, you may visit a web site that uses RealAudio plug-ins for music, speech, or a mixture of the two. RealAudio will allow you to hear musical sound while a file is being downloaded. If you are using Internet Explorer, the RealAudio plug-in is bundled with it. However, if you are using NetScape or any other browser, you can download the player software from this web site:

<http://www.realaudio.com>

. . . and install it on your computer. Another useful plug-in is Adobe's Acrobat Reader – a PDF (portable document format) reader that enables you to view elaborate electronic documents stored in PDF format:

<http://www.adobe.com/products/acrobat/readstep.html>.

Question 5   what is a cache and how does it work?

Answer: When logging on to NetScape on your college network to surf the net, you might see a dialogue box with a message asking if you want the system to maximize your cache. I suggest you click on the YES button. Cache temporarily stores the information on a page in your computer. The first time you ask for a page, your browser retrieves the page from the network. No pages are permanently stored in a cache. If you request a page you have seen before, your browser checks to see if the page is available in a cache. For example, if you use the BACK button on your browser to display a page, a cache can display the page more quickly than the network can retransmit it.

Question 6   what should I know about firewalls?

Answer: Data security and privacy is extremely important in health care. Using a firewall it is possible to protect one or more computers with Internet connections from access by external computers connected to the Internet. A firewall is a network configuration, created by software and hardware, that forms a boundary between networked computers within the firewall from those outside the firewall. The computers within the firewall become a secure subset with internal access capabilities and shared resources not available to the computers on the outside. A firewall is commonly used to protect information such as data files within an organization site. A firewall reduces the risk of intrusion by unauthorized people from the Internet. However, the same security measures can limit or require special software for those inside the firewalls who wish to access information on the outside.

Question 7   should anyone give out a credit card number on the internet?

Answer: At some point on your course you will need to buy books. While busy surfing, you may arrive at an Internet bookshop where you decide to order a book but wonder whether it is safe to make the payment using your credit card. Stop for a moment and consider how you use your credit or debit card in the 'real world'. For example, do you always ask for the copy after signing for a credit card purchase? The truth is, card numbers are so easy to steal. Stealing credit card numbers over the net is much harder, because it takes a lot of effort and technical know-how. One credit number is unlikely to warrant the effort. Nevertheless, to make the hacker's job even more difficult, most web sites at which you can use your credit card run on secure servers. Furthermore, NetScape allows you to enter your credit card number on a secure (https) NetScape Navigator form for it to be transmitted over the Internet to a secure server without the risk of an intermediary obtaining your credit card information. NetScape clearly states that 'the security features offered by NetScape

Communications technology prevent fraud that could otherwise occur as information passes through Internet computers'.

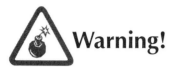

Warning!

However, before you enter into any commercial transaction over the net, be sure you are willing to trust the server administrator with your credit card number in the same way as you would if you were telling someone your credit card number over the telephone.

Question 8 what is home highway and how does it work?

Answer: Whilst your standard phone line uses analogue technology, Home Highway – a new service from BT – uses digital ISDN2e technology to give you flexibility and speed. Home Highway upgrades your existing standard telephone line by transforming it into two lines, each of which can be used for analogue and digital access simultaneously. The digital signal is far clearer than an analogue signal, allowing for greatly improved performance when using a computer. According to BT (1998)[24] '[with Home Highway] digital computer access is over four times faster than an analogue modem operating at 28.8K and can usually connect in a few seconds compared to the 45 seconds it can take using an analogue modem'. With Home Highway, you have access to unique multi-tasking opportunities at an increased speed, such as:

- A blistering 128K speed when browsing the Internet and downloading stuff
- A 64K speed on one line whilst making and receiving phone calls on the other
- A 64K speed when using two PCs to work on the Internet at the same time
- The flexibility of 64K speed for surfing the net with your PC while simultaneously using your phone for making and receiving calls or faxes.

For more Information on Home Highway, such as equipment, installation, charges, and other Q&A, pay a visit to the BT homepage at:

http://www.bthomehighway.bt.com/

. . . or call a BT adviser on Freefone 0800 222 444.

Question 9 what are trolls?

Answer: A troll is a posting deliberately intended to provoke a flame war in newsgroups. The term 'troll' has its root in fishing: 'trolling' is casting a bait a long way out and pulling it slowly back in order to attract the fish to your boat. In a similar way, trolling can gather a collection of newcomers to newsgroups and then slowly takes them to task. Here is an example of a troll. It is well known that the 'H' in 'Margaret H. Thatcher' stands for 'Hilda'. Now, if someone comes along who insists until he is blue in the face that it stands for 'Hilary' you'd want to put him right, correct? Wrong. That's what he wants. If you dare get involved, you will be rising to the bait.

Question 10 what is spamming?

Answer: This is a net expression for sending the same message to multiple newsgroups or e-mail recipients regardless of their interest (or lack of it). Most spamming consists of unsolicited advertisements. Apart from the personal aggravation it causes, spamming is also a massive waste of *bandwidth*. Russell (1998)[25] relates an interesting case of spamming that ought to serve as a warning to all of us:

Cantor and Seigal was a firm of US lawyers who went in for one of the less nice legal scams in recent years. It's not very well-known that the United States runs a Green Card lottery every year. Anyone can go along to the US embassy, fill in a card with their name and address, and every year or so they make a draw . . . the few people whose cards are drawn (from the thousands submitted) are given a Green Card – that is, full US citizenship. In the last few years, some firms of lawyers have exploited this by offering their services to 'help you get US citizenship' – that is, they will charge you £100 to fill in a card for you and put it in on your behalf. You sometimes see adverts for these services in the small ads in the back of newspapers. Cantor and Seigal took this to extremes, by putting out their advert on the Internet. In particular, they sent a copy to every single newsgroup.

This act is regarded as spamming and it is frowned on. Now, there are two possible ways of dealing with this sort of behaviour. First, you can put a complaint to their Internet Service Provider or System Administrator. Second, you can use a technique called 'mail bombing', i.e. you send an e-mail containing a very large meaningless attachment file to the perpetrators of the spam. If the volume is large enough it will cause the Internet Service Provider's system to crash. According to Russell (1998) this is exactly what happened to Cantor and Seigal. A large volume of abusive e-mail was sent to Cantor and Seigal putting their Internet Service Provider's system out of action for several days. Cantor and Seigal's account was cancelled and they were sued for damages by their Service Provider.

So there you have it!

Question 11 what are cyber cafés?

Answer: In the last couple of years, a few cafés and pubs, besides offering tea, coffee, beer, and so on, have started making available to their clients computers with Internet access. Users are charged a fee per hour to use the computers to access the Internet, and very often it is necessary for you to book time in advance (especially at lunch times, evenings and weekends).

Here is a selective list of UK Cyber Cafés:

- 3W Café at 4 Market Place, Bracknell, Berkshire
- Cyberia Caféž at 39 Whitfield Street, London
- Electric Frog at 42–44 Cockburn Street, Edinburgh
- Planet 13 at 25 High Cross Street, St Austell, Cornwall
- Revelations at Shaftesbury Square, Belfast
- The Edge at St George's Centre, St Ann's Road, Harrow, Middlesex
- Punters Cyber Café at 111 Arundel Street, Sheffield
- CyberZone at 1 Dingwall Road, Croydon, Surrey
- Chaucer Cyberspace at Chaucer Tech. School, Spring Lane, Canterbury, Kent.

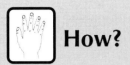
how to find more answers to questions?
There are several web sites that have a section called FAQ (Frequently Asked Questions). Here are two web sites that will give you answers to many questions you may care to ask:

* http://www.columbia.edu./cu/healthwise/alice.html
* http://www.patents.com/weblaw.sht

Question 12 what about copyright law and the net?

Answer: Copyright law usually gives the owner the exclusive right to control copying of a writing, recording, picture, or electronic transcription. When it comes to Cyberspace, the law is frustratingly vague and difficult to interpret. But to avoid copyright infringement here are a few points that net surfers should keep in mind:

* Almost everything you produce yourself on the net is protected under copyright law. As soon as you have written your work, e.g. e-mail message, posting to newsgroups, or a web creation, it's automatically copyrighted (without the need to send it anywhere, or even put a copyright notice on it). However, having a copyright symbol on your page leaves no one in any doubt.
* Copyright law does not mean that you cannot use another's work for inspiration, but simply that you are not allowed to copy it without permission. Do remember though, ideas, facts, titles, names, or short phrases are not copyrighted.
* A message to a newsgroup is under copyright, but as it was posted to a discussion list, the writer gave an implicit licence for others to quote the person in their response.
* Linking your homepage to someone else's is becoming a common practice. There does not appear to be a problem in this area as long as you do not try to take credit for the other person's work. By being on the web, there is an implied permission for others to add a link. You are not legally required to inform the web site that you are adding to his/her homepage, although this would be good netiquette. However, it is not permissible to use someone's actual list of links if that list demonstrates some originality.
* Provided images and graphics on the web are in the **Public Domain**, it is legal to use them. Otherwise, you must obtain permission from the copyright holder.
* There is a lot of excellent material on the Internet that is Public Domain and free for anyone to copy and use. However, unless the right to copy is implicit or the author has made it explicitly free to copy ('you are free to use this material'), you will be wise to keep your hands off. (The law here is somewhat fuzzy.)

Public Domain is material that, for whatever reason, is not protected by copyright law and can be used freely without permission. An example is a copyright that has expired.

Finally the law in Cyberspace is continuously evolving. To help you keep yourself up to date here are four web sites:

- 10 Big Myths About Copyright Explained
  http://www.clari.net/brad/copymyths.html

- Web Law FAQ
  http://www.patents.com/weblaw.sht

- Cyberspace Law for Non-lawyers
  http://www.lawnewsnetwork.com

- The Copyright Website
  http://www.benedict.com/

appendices

Here is a summary of typical User agreement that you can expect from colleges or universities when you register to use computing facilities. Following registration, you are given an account, i.e. a username and password. Acceptance of this account implies that you implicitly agree to comply with the college regulations governing the use of computing facilities. The full text of these 'Regulations for the Use of the Computing Service' may be issued to you and/or may be displayed in computing laboratories and in other places, e.g. students' notice board. It is your responsibility to read these regulations and to ensure that you comply with them, as any breach will render you liable to disciplinary action.

- These rules apply to anyone using any kind of computer hardware or software at the college for any purpose, even if it is their own equipment and even if it is only connected to the college through a network or telephone line. They also apply to anyone here using the computer facilities of another university or college.
- You are required to register, or be registered, in order to use college computing facilities. Any user identification or password you are given is for you alone: do not tell anyone your registration details and do not attempt to use anyone else's. If you leave the college or change your course you must tell User Services.
- Special permission is needed to use computers for personal, commercial or outside work use. There may be charges for some types of computer use.
- You must ensure that you know how to use the equipment. Follow the instructions for starting and finishing sessions and while you are using computing equipment.
- You must not damage, interfere with, or change any hardware or software; if you do you will be charged with the cost of putting it right. You need permission to move anything or to connect any new hardware. Only use authorized software. You may not load new software without permission. Do not introduce, or risk introducing, computer viruses or anything similar. Do not interfere with other users or their data or software.
- You must not create, bring in, display, produce, or circulate any offensive material.
- Smoking, eating and drinking near computing equipment may cause damage and is not allowed.
- Old data and uncollected printouts may be removed by housekeeping procedures. Do not rely on them being retained for you.
- The college does not accept responsibility for any loss caused by your use of computing facilities.
- Any breach of these Regulations may also constitute a breach of criminal or civil law but will certainly render you liable to disciplinary action.

Reproduced by kind permission of Computing Services, Canterbury Christ Church University College

Internet Service Providers (ISPs) are companies that provide you with access to the Internet by connecting (or 'dialling in') to their computers via a modem. These days ISPs can be roughly divided into three types:

- **Online (subscription) services** – They charge for the service and phone calls and often provide content.
- **'0800' ISPs** – Here you pay a fixed fee for the service and get unlimited access in return.
- **'Free' Local ISPs** (also called 'pay-as-you-go') – These are probably the best to start off with as they don't charge for their service but do make you pay for the phone calls, usually at local rates, via your phone bill.

Each has its advantages – those which charge for the service and the phonecalls tend to have a better service than the 'free' ISPs, while the '0800' ISPs tend to have been so overwhelmed by demand that their service is often quite poor, and you can find yourself struggling to get and keep online. Having said that, you may be able to find a few 'free' ISPs that provide a better service than the paid-for services. The best way to find out the truth is to experience it for yourself.

2.1 online (subscription) services and 0800

Note Information about service providers is subject to change. Details given here are for guidance only and were accurate at time of compilation. Inclusion does not imply endorsement.

Here is a selected list of the online services available, with a brief discussion of the first four. You will find a comprehensive list in most Internet magazines. All the companies on the list will provide you (on request) with free software you can subscribe to. Remember that these companies will charge you for the service and phone calls. Do not forget to ask them for details of subscription schemes on offer and do read the small print. Also, Read Subsection 2.3.5 if you have not already done so. Furthermore, it is recommended that you browse each service before committing yourself.

Table A2.1
Online (subscription) services and 0800

ISP	Web address	Contact	More information
Affinity Surf	http://www.affinity.uk.com	0870 6070792	Fifteen e-mail addresses, 10Mb web space, 50p per minute for technical support. BT Surftime site.
AOL Flat rate	http://www.aol.co.uk	0800 3765432 0800 2791234	Seven e-mail addresses, 35mb webspace, free technical support £14.99 per month for unmetered access.
Big Blue Sky	http://www.bigbluesky.uk.net	01555 888900	One-mail address, no web space, cost for technical support TBA. £25 per year for free call access.
BT Internet (Anytime)	http://www.btinternet.com	0800 800001	BT's unmetered service with free calls all the time. Very popular, but lots of complaints. Five e-mail addresses, 10mb webspace, 50p per minute technical support.
BT SurfTime	http://www.btsurftime.co.uk	Online	A BT system that runs alongside a range of ISPs.
Calenet	http://www.calenet.co.uk	07050 687211	Unlimited e-mail addresses, 15Mb webspace, national rate for technical support. £39 per year for free access.
ClaraNet (Free time Anytime)	http://www.claranet.co.uk	0845 3551000	Unlimited e-mail addresses, 50mb webspace, local rate for technical support. £5.99 per month for 12 hours of free access. BT phone line needed.
CompuServe 2000	http://www.compuserve.co.uk	0870 6000800	Seven e-mail addresses, 10mb webspace, national rate for technical support. £7.50 per month (pay ISP)+ plus call at local rate. First month's subscription free.
Demon Internet	http://www.demon.net	0845 2722999	Unlimited e-mail addresses, 20mb webspace, local rate for technical support. £11.75 per month (Pay ISP)
Easynet	http://www.easydial.co.uk	0845 3334000	Unlimited e-mail addresses, unlimited webspace, local rate for technical support. £11.99 per month (pay ISP).
Excite	http://www.excite.co.uk	Online	One e-mail address, 5Mb webspace, £1 per minute for technical support. £89.99 per year free access (one hour cut off).
Freechariot	http://www.freechariot.net	Online	Web based e-mail, 50Mb webspace, 25p per minute for technical support. £14.49 per month for free access.
PurpleDial	http://www.purplenet.co.uk	0800 7834535	Unlimited e-mail addresses, 25mb webspace, local rate for technical support. £7.50 per month for free access.

ISP	Web address	Contact	More information
Freedom2Surf (Anytime)	http://www.freedom2surf.net	Online 01727 811530	Unlimited e-mail addresses, 20Mb webspace, local rate for technical support. £9.40 per month for free access.
Freeserve (Anytime)	http://www.freeserve.com)	0870 8720099	Unlimited e-mail addresses, 15Mb webspace, 50p for technical support. The UK's most popular ISP. You need a BT phoneline for the unmetered service.
Genie Internet	http://www.genie.co.uk	0906 3020220	Five e-mail addresses, 25Mb webspace, 50p per minute for technical support. £14.99 a month for free access (BT Internet anytime).
NetScalibur	http://www.dircon.net	0800 0720000	Unlimited e-mail addresses, 20Mb webspace, local rate for technical support. From £4.99 a month (pay ISP).
Strayduck	http://www.strayduck.com	0906 6199000	Unlimited e-mail addresses, 25Mb webspace, 50p per minute for technical support. From £14.99 a month for free access.
Tiny Online	http://www.tinyconnect.co.uk	Online	Five e-mail addresses, 15Mb webspace, 50p per minute for technical support. From £25.99 a month for free call access (£6.99 for off peak).
U-Net	http://www.u-net.net	0845 3308000	Unlimited e-mail addresses, 25Mb webspace, local rate for technical support. £12 per month (pay ISP).

The main point to remember here is that you will be paying up to £1 per minute for calls to the companies when you need technical help. If you are unlikely to get stuck then there is nothing to worry about.

Table A2.2
Free internet service providers ('pay-as-you-go')

ISP	Web address	Contact	More information
4TheNet	http://www.4thenet.co.uk	Online	Unlimited e-mail addresses, unlimited web space, £1 per minute for technical support.
Abel Gratis	http://www.abelgratis.co.uk		Unlimited e-mail addresses, 50Mb web space, 25p per minute for technical support.
Barclay Bank	http://www.is.barclays.co.uk	0800 494949	Five e-mail addresses, no web space, 3p weekends, 8p weekdays for technical support.
BigWig	http://www.bigwig.net	0870 7401033	Seven e-mail addresses, 15Mb web space, £1 per minute for technical support.
Blue Carrots	http://www.bluecarrots.com	Online	Five e-mail addresses, 20Mb web space, 50p per minute for technical support.
British Library	http://www.britishlibrary.net	01937 546585	Unlimited e-mail addresses, 2–20Mb web space, 50p per minute for technical support.
Care4Free	http://www.care4free.net	0870 6066334	Charity based. Five e-mail addresses, 15Mb web space, 50p per minute for technical support.
Connect Free	http://www.connectfree	0870 742111	Unlimited e-mail addresses, unlimited web space, 50p per minute for technical support.
Dabsol	http://www.dabsol.co.uk	Online	Unlimited e-mail addresses, unlimited web space, 49/39p per minute for technical support.
Doctors Net	http://www.doctors.net.uk	Online	Doctors only. One e-mail address, 3Mb web space, local rate for technical support.
Euphony Net	http://www.euphony.net	0118 9218500	Unlimited e-mail addresses, unlimited web space, 50p per minute for technical support.
Free Online	http://www.free-online.net	0870 7060504	Five e-mail addresses, unlimited web space, national rate for technical support.

ISP	Web address	Contact	More information
FreecallUK	http://www.freecall-uk.co.uk	Online	Five e-mail addresses, no web space yet, 50p per minute for technical support.
Freeola	http://www.freeola.net	Online	Unlimited e-mail addresses, unlimited web space, national rate for technical support.
Freeserve (no ties)	http://www.freeserve.com	0870 8720090	Unlimited e-mail addresses, 15Mb web space, 50p per minute for technical support. Access at local rates. The most popular ISP, usually reliable.
FreeUK	http://www.freeuk.net	08453 555555	Unlimited e-mail addresses, 25Mb web space, 50p per minute for technical support.
IC24	http://www.ic24.net	0906 7444222	Five e-mail addresses, 10Mb web space, 50p per minute for technical support.
ICOM43	http://www.icom43.net	0906 7522022	Unlimited e-mail addresses, 15Mb web space, 75p per minute for technical support.
ICScotland net	http://www.icscotland.net	0906 7444222	Five e-mail addresses, 10Mb web space, 50p per minute for technical support. Also free calls evenings and weekends.
LineOne	http://www.lineone.net	0906 3020100	Five e-mail addresses, 50Mb web space, 50p per minute for technical support.
MSN Freeweb	http://www.msn.co.uk	0870 601 10000	Web-based e-mail, no web space, national rate for technical support.
NatWest Com	http://www.natwest.com	0906 302333	Web-based e-mail, no web space, 50p per minute for technical support.
Netscape Online	http://www.netscapeonline.co.uk	0800 9230009	Unlimited e-mail addresses, 20Mb web space, 50p per minute for technical support.
Orange Net	http://www.orange.net	0906 7162626	One e-mail address, 15Mb web space, 50p per minute for technical support.

Table A2.2 *(cont.)*

ISP	Web address	Contact	More information
Oxfam	http://www.oxfam.org.uk	0870 2410874	Web-based e-mail, no web space, 50p per minute for technical support. Charity based.
PlusNet	http://www.plus.net	0870 7058000	Unlimited e-mail addresses, unlimited web space, national rate for technical support.
Supanet	http://www.supanet.com	0906 715155	Unlimited e-mail addresses, 15Mb web space, 50p per minute for technical support.
Surf&Save	http://www.pgen.net	0900 2909158	Five e-mail addresses, 10Mb web space, national rate for technical support. Save money on electricity.
TESCO Net	http://www.tesco.net	0906 3020111	Five e-mail addresses, 10Mb web space, 50p per minute for technical support.
The Mutual Net	http://www.themutual.net	0906 3003366	Two e-mail addresses, 25Mb web space, 50p per minute for technical support.
Totalise	http://www.totalise.net	0800 5427566	Unlimited e-mail addresses, 20Mb web space, free technical support.
UK Online	http://www.ukonline.co.uk	0906 296555	Unlimited e-mail addresses, unlimited web space, 25p per minute for technical support.
UnisonFree.Net	http://www.unisonfree.net	0906 2965599	Unlimited e-mail addresses, unlimited web space, 25p per minute for technical support.
Virgin. Net	http://www.virgin.net	0845 6500000 0500 558800	Five e-mail addresses, 10Mb web space, £1.00 or £5.99 monthly for technical support.
Waitrose	http://www.waitrose.com	0800 3767060	Five e-mail addresses, 10Mb web space, local rate for technical support.
Waterstones	http://www.waterstones.yahoo.co.uk	0906 3021200	Web-based e-mail address, no web space, 50p per minute for technical support.
WH Smith Online	http://www.whsmith.co.uk	0906 3020001	Unlimited e-mail addresses, 12Mb web space, 50p per minute for technical support.
World Online	http://www.worldonline.co.uk	0906 7113311	Unlimited e-mail addresses, 12Mb web space, 50p per minute for technical support. Also a fixed fee per month for 100 free hours.

A standard modem connection is 56K. Any Internet connection that offers bandwidth that's higher than 56K is referred to as 'broadband'. This can include the likes of ADSL (Asymmetric Digital Subscriber Line), ISDN (Integrated Services Digital Network) and cable. The main benefit is that in some cases the speed could be ten times faster than a standard analogue modem. Thus, file transfer times are significantly faster. This is particularly useful where multimedia applications are involved. With a broadband connection, multimedia content like audio and video can be delivered smoothly and seamlessly to your PC with TV-quality pictures and CD-quality sound.

- **ADSL** – This is the next great leap in the world of Internet communications. It is up to ten times faster than your existing modem connection and it is 'always on'. Once you have established connection you can stay online for as long as you like. There are no call cost when using the Internet, all you pay is the fixed monthly fee. Also you can still use your phone to make and receive calls while you are connected. You need to be a BT customer with an ordinary phone line in order to take advantage of this service. There are other ISPs offering an ADSL service (see Table A2.3 below).
- **Cable** – Also around ten times faster than your standard dial-up connection. You need to have cable in order to take advantage of this service. Like ADSL, it is always on and you can make and receive phone calls while online.
- **Wireless** – Here there is no need for a cable modem or an ADSL link because the broadband connection to the Internet is made via an aerial on your roof and an indoor unit or 'Speedbox' which connect directly to your PC.

Table A2.3
Broadband
services (no call costs)

ISP	Web address	Contact	More information
Blueyonder	http://www.blueyonder.co.uk	0800 9530454	Five e-mail addresses, 30Mb web space, free technical support (morning only). Superfast cable access, Only £25 per month if included with other Telewest services.
Btopenworld	http://www.btopenworld.co.uk	0800 1696922	One e-mail address, 20Mb web space, free technical support. Fast ADSL connection.
Ntl128k	http://www.ntl.co.uk	0800 0522000	Five e-mail addresses, 10Mb web space, local for technical support. New semi-broadband service. Faster than dial-up.
Ntl512k	http://www.ntl.co.uk	0800 0522000	Five e-mail addresses, 10Mb web space, free technical support. Winners of Future Internet Award for best broadband ISP. Good service. Good price.
PlusNet Home ADSL	http://www.plus.net	0845 1400200	Unlimited e-mail addresses, 250Mb web space, local rate for technical support. Up to 40 times faster than an ordinary dial-up connection, with free .co.uk domain.

Here is a list showing the countries which have access to the Internet or general e-mail services. The country codes[26] have been derived from *The World Factbook 2002*. These are the two letters that you can expect to find at the end of World Wide Web domain names.

Table A3.1
The following countries have Internet connection

Country code	Country	Country code	Country
.ad	Andorra	.cm	Cameroon
.ae	United Arab Emirates	.cn	China
.af	Afghanistan	.co	Colombia
.ag	Antigua and Barbuda	.cr	Costa Rica
.ai	Anguilla	.cs	Czechoslovakia (former)
.al	Albania	.cu	Cuba
.am	Armenia	.cv	Cape Verde
.an	Netherlands Antilles	.cx	Christmas Island
.ao	Angola	.cy	Cyprus
.aq	Antarctica	.cz	Czech Republic
.ar	Argentina	.de	Germany
.as	American Samoa	.dj	Djibouti
.at	Austria	.dk	Denmark
.au	Australia	.dm	Dominica
.aw	Aruba	.do	Dominican Republic
.az	Azerbaijan	.dz	Algeria
.ba	Bosnia and Herzegovina	.ec	Ecuador
.bb	Barbados	.ee	Estonia
.bd	Bangladesh	.eg	Egypt
.be	Belgium	.eh	Western Sahara
.bf	Burkina Faso	.er	Eritrea
.bg	Bulgaria	.es	Spain
.bh	Bahrain	.et	Ethiopia
.bi	Burundi	.fi	Finland
.bj	Benin	.fj	Fiji
.bm	Bermuda	.fk	Falkland Islands (Malvinas)
.bn	Brunei Darussalam	.fm	Micronesia
.bo	Bolivia	.fo	Faroe Islands
.br	Brazil	.fr	France
.bs	Bahamas	.fx	France, Metropolitan
.bt	Bhutan	.ga	Gabon
.bv	Bouvet Island	.gb	Great Britain (UK)
.bw	Botswana	.gd	Grenada
.by	Belarus	.ge	Georgia
.bz	Belize	.gf	French Guiana
.ca	Canada	.gh	Ghana
.cc	Cocos (Keeling) Islands	.gi	Gibraltar
.cf	Central African Republic	.gl	Greenland
.cg	Congo	.gm	Gambia
.ch	Switzerland	.gn	Guinea
.ci	Cote d'Ivoire (Ivory Coast)	.gp	Guadeloupe
.ck	Cook Islands	.gq	Equatorial Guinea
.cl	Chile	.gr	Greece

Country code	Country	Country code	Country
.gs	South Georgia and South Sandwich Islands	.ls	Lesotho
		.lt	Lithuania
.gt	Guatemala	.lu	Luxembourg
.gu	Guam	.lv	Latvia
.gw	Guinea-Bissau	.ly	Libya
.gy	Guyana	.ma	Morocco
.hk	Hong Kong	.mc	Monaco
.hm	Heard and McDonald Islands	.md	Moldova
		.mg	Madagascar
.hn	Honduras	.mh	Marshall Islands
.hr	Croatia (Hrvatska)	.mk	Macedonia
.ht	Haiti	.ml	Mali
.hu	Hungary	.mm	Myanmar
.id	Indonesia	.mn	Mongolia
.ie	Ireland	.mo	Macau
.il	Israel	.mp	Northern Mariana Islands
.in	India	.mq	Martinique
.io	British Indian Ocean Territory	.mr	Mauritania
		.ms	Montserrat
.iq	Iraq	.mt	Malta
.ir	Iran	.mu	Mauritius
.is	Iceland	.mv	Maldives
.it	Italy	.mw	Malawi
.jm	Jamaica	.mx	Mexico
.jo	Jordan	.my	Malaysia
.jp	Japan	.mz	Mozambique
.ke	Kenya	.na	Namibia
.kg	Kyrgyzstan	.nc	New Caledonia
.kh	Cambodia	.ne	Niger
.ki	Kiribati	.nf	Norfolk Island
.km	Comoros	.ng	Nigeria
.kn	Saint Kitts and Nevis	.ni	Nicaragua
.kp	Korea (North)	.nl	Netherlands
.kr	Korea (South)	.no	Norway
.kw	Kuwait	.np	Nepal
.ky	Cayman Islands	.nr	Nauru
.kz	Kazakhstan	.nt	Neutral Zone
.la	Laos	.nu	Niue
.lb	Lebanon	.nz	New Zealand (Aotearoa)
.lc	Saint Lucia	.om	Oman
.li	Liechtenstein	.pa	Panama
.lk	Sri Lanka	.pe	Peru
.lr	Liberia	.pf	French Polynesia

Table A3.1 (*cont.*)

Country code	Country	Country code	Country
.pg	Papua New Guinea	.tp	East Timor
.ph	Philippines	.tr	Turkey
.pk	Pakistan	.tt	Trinidad and Tobago
.pl	Poland	.tv	Tuvalu
.pm	St Pierre and Miquelon	.tw	Taiwan
.pn	Pitcairn	.tz	Tanzania
.pr	Puerto Rico	.ua	Ukraine
.pt	Portugal	.ug	Uganda
.pw	Palau	.uk	United Kingdom
.py	Paraguay	.um	US Minor Outlying Islands
.qa	Qatar	.us	United States
.re	Reunion	.uy	Uruguay
.ro	Romania	.uz	Uzbekistan
.ru	Russia	.va	Vatican City State (Holy
.rw	Rwanda		See)
.sa	Saudi Arabia	.vc	St Vincent and the
.sb	Solomon Islands		Grenadines
.sc	Seychelles	.ve	Venezuela
.sd	Sudan	.vg	Virgin Islands (British)
.se	Sweden	.vi	Virgin Islands (US)
.sg	Singapore	.vn	Viet Nam
.sh	St Helena	.vu	Vanuatu
.si	Slovenia	.wf	Wallis and Futuna Islands
.sj	Svalbard and Jan Mayen	.ws	Samoa
	Islands	.ye	Yemen
.sk	Slovak Republic	.yt	Mayotte
.sl	Sierra Leone	.yu	Yugoslavia
.sm	San Marino	.za	South Africa
.sn	Senegal	.zm	Zambia
.so	Somalia	.zr	Zaire
.sr	Tunisia	.zw	Zimbabwe
.to	Tonga		

Unfortunately, there will be times when you try to visit a web site and instead you receive strange error messages. There is no point getting too worked-up about it. Just accept them as part of the magic of the net. Here are some of the most common NetScape Navigator error messages, with suggested actions.

Table A4.1

Error message	Meaning
400- Bad request	It may be that you have not typed the URL correctly. • Check the URL for errors, such as upper or lower case letters, colons, forward slashes.
401- Unauthorised	You're attempting to enter a forbidden site, or you've entered an incorrect password. • If you do have access, try the site again, ensuring that you type your password correctly.
403- Forbidden	If you are not entitled to access a site or a certain document, then there isn't a lot you can do other than trying again at a later date.
404- Not found	It is most likely that you have typed the address incorrectly. It is also possible that the page has moved or is no longer available. • Try typing the address again.
503- Service unavailable	The web site may be down for a variety of reasons. • Try the site again at a later time or date.
File contains no data	It is possible that the document is being updated just as you tried to access it. • Try again later.
Host unavailable	You are probably trying to access a site that is down for maintenance. • Try again later.
Connection refused by host	You are trying to access a secure document without proper authority. • If you think you have the right to that document, contact the site's Webmaster.
Unable to locate the server	You are using an incorrect URL, or the server does not exist anymore. • If you are sure you have the correct URL, check that you are entering it correctly.
Network connection was refused by the server	The server is probably busy. Try again later.
Too many users	The site is very busy. • Try again later.
Unable to locate host	You have probably lost connection or the web site is down. • Try clicking the **Reload** button on the toolbar

Access code is a unique combination of characters, usually letters or numbers, used in communications as identification for gaining access to a computer. The access code is generally referred to as Username or user ID and password. (Read Subsection 2.1.1)

Account is a term used in computer science to describe a record-keeping arrangement employed by a System Manager at a college, university or health organization, and a Vendor of an online service. It helps Vendors to identify their subscribers, for example, for billing. System Managers of multi-user systems use it to identify their users for administration and security purposes. A personal computing account is rather like your bank account; this has a Password that 'only' you know, together with an account name (*Username*) that identifies you. (Read Section 2.1)

Adobe Acrobat is a software package that allows you to view electronic documents, which have been stored in .pdf format. (See .pdf)

Anonymous FTP Some FTP sites are called Anonymous because the system does not need to find out who you are before letting you in. You can log in to these sites by entering the word *Anonymous* for *Username* and for password you enter your e-mail address or simply type the word *guess*. (Read Subsection 7.1.1)

Application A program that performs a specific task such as word processing, database management or web browsing.

Archie is an older system that was and can still be used to quickly find files that are located on the FTP sites. (Read Section 7.2)

Archie servers are located around the Internet. It can help you find the exact location of the files you are looking for literally in seconds. These servers keep track of all the *anonymous FTP* public files on the Internet by searching the public directories of the FTP hosts on a regular basis and maintaining a list of all files.

Articles see *posting*

Bandwidth is a general term for the amount of information that can be transferred over an Internet connection.

BIOME An Internet search service for Health and Life Sciences. It is part of the RDN – the UK's national Internet search service designed for academics and professionals – built with funding from the government and national research councils.

Bookmark A way of storing web addresses so you can find them easily (Bookmarks can be found on NetScape – they are called 'Favorites' on Microsoft Internet Explorer). (Read Subsection 3.2.3)

Boolean searching A technique for expanding or refining searches when searching a database using the Boolean operators AND, OR, NOT to link keywords. (Read Subsection 4.2.1)

Bounce means to return undeliverable. If you mail a message to a bad address, it bounces back to your mailbox. Conversely, if your e-mail address is erroneous, when people attempt to reply to your message it bounces back to their mailbox. (Read Subsection 5.3.2)

Browser is a computer program that enables you to view web pages on the Internet. Although the NetScape browser is a very popular program, its main competitor is Microsoft Internet Explorer. The main advantage of this application is that Microsoft gives it away for free, while NetScape is a commercial software package. There are things that NetScape can do and Internet Explorer can't, and vice versa, but in general they are equally powerful. (Read Subsections: 3.1.3, 3.1.4, 3.2.1)

CD-ROM This stands for 'Compact Disc Read-Only Memory', which is a disk used for storing and distributing large volumes of data. (Read Subsection 2.3.1)

Click A single press and release of a mouse button (see double-click).

Clipboard This allows data to be copied within and between *applications* in *Windows*, i.e. when you use the 'Cut and Paste' options in Windows.

Computer network is a set of interconnected computer systems, terminals, and communications equipment.

Cookies are small text-files that some web sites store on your computer so that they know who you are next time you visit. (Read Question 2 in Twelve Big Questions and Answers.)

Cursor is a movable, blinking bar of light on a VDU screen marking the next point of character entry or change.

Data These are facts, numbers, letters and symbols stored in a computer.

Database can be described as a sophisticated electronic filing cabinet capable of storing and sorting large amounts of data in an organized manner. The data can be accessed quickly.

Desktop is a computer that is kept on top of a desk or any suitable hard work surface.

Dot matrix is a fairly basic, but flexible printer. It can produce text or graphics in the form of a matrix of small dots, with each character formed by a series of pins striking a ribbon. They are generally used for jobs where the quality of the printing is not crucial.

Double-click This is clicking a mouse button twice in quick succession.

Download is to copy files (of any type) to your own computer from some other computer. The opposite term is to *upload*.

Electronic journal A journal which is available electronically. It may be available in electronic format only, or it may have a print equivalent. Some are available free of charge, others require payment or a subscription. (Read Section 3.3 Journals for health professionals.)

Electronic mail or e-mail is essentially a text system that allows messages to be passed from one user to reach another user who is connected to the Internet or a computer network. (Read Unit 5.)

Error message A textual message displayed when the computer detects a problem. (Read Appendix 4.)

FAQ This is short for 'Frequently Asked Questions' – either a frequently asked question, or a list of frequently asked questions. FAQs are commonly used on the web to offer novice users help on a particular topic. (Read Twelve Big Questions and Answers.)

Favorites A way of storing web addresses so you can find them easily. Favourites can be found on Microsoft Internet Explorer – they are called 'Bookmarks' on NetScape. (Read Subsection 3.2.3)

File A collection of related *data* or records. A file is used to store data, or program, on disk for later use.

Firewall A security device that prevents intruders from entering a private network. (Read Question 6 in Twelve Big Questions and Answers)

Flame Abusive message posted to a newsgroup as part of an on going argument.

Freeware Software distributed via the Internet that can be downloaded and utilized for free.

FTP stands for File Transfer Protocol. It is a method of transferring files from one computer to another over the net. (Read Section 7.1)

Full Text When it is possible to view a complete document, rather than simply a summary or abstract of it.

Full-duplex A full-duplex card can record your voice while playing the incoming voice. This enables both of you to talk at the same time (ideal for discussions). With half-duplex you can either talk or listen, but not both.

.gif GIF is short for 'Graphics Interchange Format', which is the name of a computer file format for images. So if you see a file called something like 'game.gif' the chances are it will be a computer graphic of a game!

Gateway A program or device that acts as a kind of translator between two networks that wouldn't otherwise be able to communicate with each other.

Gopher is an older system that lets you find text information by using menus. (Read Section 7.3)

Hacker is a term normally used to describe a skilled programmer who invades systems and ferrets out information on individual computer access codes through a process of trial and error.

Hardware The tangible electronic (and mechanical) devices which constitute a computer system. This includes both the computer itself, the monitor (with the screen), the keyboard, and any peripherals.

Headers are the lines of text that appear at the beginning of every Internet mail message. (Read Subsection 5.1.2)

Hits There are two meanings: (1) search hits – the number of results retrieved from an Internet search; (2) site hits – the number of times a server receives a request for a web object such as text files, graphics, video, and so on. Not a reliable gauge to compare different sites, as one page with five graphics will register six hits when viewed, whilst a page with no graphics will display one hit.

Homepage is a term used on the Internet to refer to the first page of a web site.

Hosts are computers that are directly connected to the Internet.

HTML Hypertext mark-up language: a code used in documents to indicate how information is to be displayed on the World Wide Web. HTML files are read by a *web browser* and it interprets codes about the format and size of text and where links to other files are to be placed. (Read Section 8.1)

HTTP is short for 'Hypertext Transfer Protocol' – the standard language that World Wide Web *clients* and *servers* use to communicate. (Read Subsection 3.17)

Hypertext (hyperlink) is a system of clickable texts used on the web. These clickable texts serve as a cross reference to another part of the document (or an entirely different document). (Read Subsection 3.1.5)

Hypermedia Hyperlinks that include forms of media.

IBM (short for International Business Machines) is an American computer manufacturer, with headquarters in Armonk, New York. The company is a major supplier of information-processing products in the US and around the world. Its products are used in a wide variety of industries, including business, government, science, defence, education, medicine, and space exploration.

Icon A graphical representation of an object in a Graphical User Interface.

Inbox is a term used to describe the box that stores all your incoming mail until it is read. (Read Subsection 5.3.2)

Inkjet printers can be described as the 'poor man's' laser printers. The inkjet printing system prints characters and graphics by firing ink drops at the paper from thin nozzles. These printers use a replaceable ink cartridge that contains both the print head and the ink.

Internet can be defined as a system that lets thousands of computers all over the world talk to each other.

Intranet When a private network inside a company or organization uses the same kinds of software and technology as you would normally find on the public Internet it is commonly referred to as an intranet. For example many companies/hospitals have internal web sites that can only be accessed internally by employees or guests.

.jpeg This is short for 'Joint Photographic Experts Group', which is an identification number assigned to journals, newspapers or other serial publications.

Laser printers are fast, flexible and sophisticated. They produce high-quality printing. They work on similar principles to a photocopier, using a photo-sensitive drum, and can produce between 4 and 20 pages per minute.

Laptop is a type of computer light enough for you to use while resting it on your lap, and because it weighs around 9 to 12 pounds it can also be carried around. (Read Subsection 2.3.1)

Links are *hypertext*, identifiable by being underlined and a different colour from the ordinary text around it. Links can take you to other documents or other parts of the same document. On the web, links can appear as text or pictures. (Read Subsection 3.1.1)

List server program is a piece of software on a computer that reads the e-mail you send. For example, if you send an e-mail to subscribe to a list, it will automatically add your e-mail address to its list. For automatic lists, it is important that your e-mail request is constructed in a certain way.

Mailing list This term has two meanings: (a) a list of e-mail addresses to which you can send the same message without making endless copies of it, all with different addresses inserted; and (b) a discussion group similar to newsgroups, but all the messages sent to the group are forwarded to its members by e-mail. (Read Section 6.2)

Menu A list of options from which the user selects an action to be performed by entering a letter or moving the cursor.

Modem is a device that converts the information on a computer into sound so that it can travel down the telephone line, and once it gets to the other end, the modem converts it back again into its original form. (Read Subsection 2.3.2)

Mouse A peripheral device incorporating a ball, which is rolled around a flat surface. The movement is translated into movement of a cursor around the monitor screen.

Multimedia The combination of plain text, pictures, sound, and even moving video clips.

Netiquette The cultural and social rules on the Internet. Ignoring them may result in being *flamed* or castigated in public. (Read Section 5.5 and Subsection 6.1.5)

Network see *computer network*.

News server is a computer (or program) dedicated to transferring the contents of newsgroups around the net, and to and from your computer. This may be referred to as an NNTP server. These computers are maintained by companies, organizations and individuals, and can host thousands of newsgroups.

Newsgroup is a collection of messages posted by individuals to a news server. (Read Section 6.1)

Newsreader is the software program you use to access newsgroups, and to read, send and reply to articles. (Read Subsection 6.1.2)

OMNI This is short for 'Organizing Medical Networked Information – a medical gateway in the UK. (Read Subsection 4.1.4.2)

Online is a synonym for 'connected'. Anything connected to your computer and ready for action can be said to be online. In Internet terms it means that you have successfully dialled into your service provider's computer and are now connected to the net. The opposite term is *offline*.

OPAC is short for 'Online Public Access catalogue', a library catalogue available in electronic form.

Password is a secret code used to keep things private. (Read Subsection 2.1.1)

PC is short for 'Personal Computer' – a general term for a microcomputer designed for use by a single user at a time. (Read Subsection 2.3.1)

PDF is short for 'Portable Document Format', which is a file format for electronic documents. (Read Question 1 in Twelve Big Questions and Answers.)

Plug-in A plug-in application is a computer program used to enhance the use you get from a web browser. For example, plug-in applications can help you hear music and sounds over the web, see videos and TV over the web, see cartoon animations over the web, read documents in a set format from the web, etc.

Posting When you send an e-mail message, the word 'sending' is quite good enough. When you send a message to a *newsgroup*, it isn't. Instead, for no adequately explained reason, the word *posting* is used. The word *article* is used to describe the message itself. (Read Section 6.1)

POP3 This is the method used to retrieve e-mail messages from your Internet Service Provider's mail server. Mail accounts that support this protocol can be checked for new messages from any PC. All that is needed is a username, password and the mail server address details. (Read Section 5.8 and also look up SMTP)

Printout This refers to anything printed out by a peripheral, or any computer-generated hard copy.

Program is a collection of instructions needed to solve a particular problem or to guide the computer in its operation.

RAM An acronym for Random Access Memory. It is a temporary storage space for information you are currently working on. (Read Subsection 2.3.1)

Refresh rate is the rate the electrons scan the screen. Your computer measures this rate in hertz (Hz). The higher the rate, the better. (Read Subsection 2.3.1)

RDN This is short for 'Resource Discovery Network', an Internet search service designed for academics and professionals – the UK's centre for its national subject gateways (e.g. NMAP, OMNI, SOSIG, etc.) – built with funding from the government and national research councils.

Record A collection of related data items, e.g. the personnel record of an individual. (Read Section 4.2)

Robot A software program that crawls around the web to find, catalogue and report information it has been told to search for. Also known as agents, wanderers and spiders. (Read Subsection 4.1.3)

Scroll bars These control what is displayed in the window. The position of the scroll bar button indicates the position of the information displayed in the total workspace. For example, if the scroll bar button is in the middle of the scroll bar, there is an equal amount of information off-screen on either side.

Search engines are indexes of WWW sites built automatically by a program called a spider, a robot or a worm. These programs constantly scour the web and return with information about a page's location, titles and contents, which is then added to an index. To search for a certain type of information, you just type in keywords and the search engine will display a list of sites containing these words. Search engines have the benefit of being up to date but the downside is that if, for example, you search for viral meningitis, the resulting list won't necessarily contain information about meningitis of the viral type – some may just be pages in which the words 'viral' and 'meningitis' both happen to appear. Directories don't have this problem because they list the subject of a page rather than the words it contains, but their downside is that they won't always find the newest sites. Sites get listed in directories when their authors submit them for inclusion. See also *web directories*. (Read Subsection 4.1.3)

Server A computer which provides a service to other client computers.

Service provider is a general term for a company that gives you access to the Internet by letting you dial into its computer. This may be an Internet Service Provider (ISP) or an Online Service Provider (IOP). (Read Subsection 2.3.5)

SLIP and **PPP** (SLIP is short for Serial Line Internet Protocol and PPP is short for Point-to-Point Protocol). They are Internet standards for transmitting Internet Protocol (IP) packets over serial lines (phone lines). Internet information is packaged into IP packets, a method for enclosing data into small, transmittable units (wrapped up at one end, unbundled on the other). A service provider might offer SLIP, PPP, or both. Your computer must use connection software (usually provided by the service provider) that matches the protocol of the server's connection software. PPP is a more recent and more robust protocol than SLIP. So if you have a choice, select PPP. (Read Subsection 2.3.5)

SMTP (Short for Simple Mail Transfer Protocol). It is a method used to send e-mail. On some occasions it can also be used to receive messages. (See POP3)

Software Broadly speaking, it refers to the programs that provide the driving force of all computing systems. There are two types: operating systems software and applications software.

SOSIG is short for 'the Social Science Information Gateway' – an Internet search service for social science, business and law. (Read Subsection 4.14.3)

Spam A term used originally to mean posting a message to multiple newsgroups. Now it is used to describe unsolicited e-mail advertising. Named after a sketch on Monty Python.

Spider see *Robot*

Tag is the name for *HTML* codes added to a plain text in a document. This transforms it into a web page with full formatting and links to other files and pages. (Read Table 8.1)

Telnet is a system that lets you connect from your computer to another across the Internet and use it as if you were directly connected to that computer. A slightly different version of Telnet, developed by IBM, is known as tn3270. (Read Section 7.4)

Toolbars are bars usually running along the top of the application allowing the user to carry out functions, e.g. menu bar, title bar, formatting toolbar.

Thread is an ongoing topic of conversation in a newsgroup or *mailing list*. When someone posts a message with a new subject line they're starting a new thread. Any replies to this message and replies to replies, and so on will have the same subject line and continue the thread.

Trojan is a virus that disguises itself in the form of something else, e.g. a real program. It can damage your PC but won't replicate and forward itself to other users.

U-Net limited is one of several *Internet Service Providers* (ISP). It is a service that is aimed solely at Windows users. (For a list of other ISPs refer to Appendix 2)

Upload The process of sending a data file or program to a distant location by means of a communications channel, such as a telephone line (see also download). (Read Section 8.4)

URL (pronounced 'earl') is the unique 'address' of a file on the Internet and is short for Uniform Resource Locator.

Usenet news system is a worldwide bulletin board system, which allows you to take part in discussions on a wide range of topics and is the main public discussion space on the net.

Username is a unique name you are assigned by a service enabling you to connect to it and identify yourself, demonstrating you are entitled to access it.

VDU This is short for 'Visual Display Unit'. A combined monitor and keyboard. Also referred to as a terminal. (Read Subsection 2.3.1)

Virus Rogue program which can transfer itself from one disk to another, unbeknown to the owner of the receiving disk. (Read Section 5.9 and also Question 3 in Twelve Big Questions and Answers)

.Wav is short for 'waveform', which is a computer file format for sounds. So if you see a file called something like 'ding-dong.wav' the chances are it will be a sound file of a door bell ringing.

Web directories are hand-built lists of pages sorted into categories. Although you can search directories using a keyword search, it's often as easy to click on a category and then click your way through the ever more specific subdirectories until you find the subject you're interested in. See also search engines. (Read Subsection 4.1.2)

Webmaster The administrator responsible for the management and often design of a web site.

Web address A unique address that allows you to access a web site. An example is http://cant.ac.uk. Also called a *URL*.

Web page is a single document that can be found on the web. It can be any length, like a document in a word processor. Pages can contain text, graphics, sound and video-clips, together with clever effects and controls. A group of web pages is a web site. The first page of a web site is often called the *homepage*.

Web site is a term loosely used to refer to a group of pages on the web. A site could be a single page or several complex pages belonging to a university, college, NHS trust or a nurse therapist.

Windows is a collection of programs, or suite of programs, written for personal computers and published by Microsoft. It is sometimes referred to as a GUI (graphical user interface). There are several versions around: Windows 3.1, Windows95, Windows98, Windows ME, Windows2000, Windows NT, and Windows XP. The last is the most recent and most sophisticated.

Windows NT This is a true multitasking, multithreaded 32-bit operating system for IBM or IBM compatible PCs that are connected to a network. It has increased power and stability, but it is not quite as user friendly as Windows 95 is and it also does not support Plug & Play.

Workstation Powerful, individual computer system with keyboard, graphics monitor and mouse. PCs can be referred to as workstations but this term usually refers to more powerful, non-DOS systems.

World Wide Web (Also know as WWW, W3 or simply the web). A distributed information service based around *online* hypertext documents accessed using a web browser like NetScape or Microsoft Internet Explorer. The system was developed by an Englishman, Tim Berners-Lee, at CERN, the European Centre for Research into Particle Physics, in Switzerland.

references (vancouver system citation – see section 9.3.2)

1 Ballard, E. (1996) Getting to grips with it! – Is it worth the effort? In: *CTI Nursing and Midwifery Newsletter* 2(1): Oct. 96: pp. 12–13.

2 Howson, N. (1997). What use is the Internet to nurses? In: *CTI Nursing and Midwifery Newsletter* 3(1) Oct. 97: pp. 6–7.

3 Russell, C. (1998) *Internet UK in Easy Steps.* 3rd edition. Warwickshire: Computer Step.

4 Cooper, C. (2001) The Internet and IT for busy nurses and therapists. (WWW). Available from: <http://www.carol-cooper.ac.uk/book/> [Accessed: 22 Dec. 2002].

5 Murray, P.J. (1997) Nurses talking on-line: Who's out there and what are they saying? In: *CTI Nursing and Midwifery Newsletter* 2(3) June 1997: pp. 13–14.

6 Levine, J.R.,Young, M.L. and Reinhold, A. (2000) *The Internet for Dummies – Quick Reference.* 6th edition. Forster City: IDG Books Worldwide Inc.

7 Howson, N. (1998) ScHARRP-eyed: What use is the Internet for nurses? Keeping current on the net. In: *CTI Nursing and Midwifery Newsletter* 3(3) June 98, pp. 12–13.

8 Harmon, C. (1996) *Using the Internet Online Services and CD-ROMs for Writing Research and Term Papers.* New York: Neal-Schuman Publishers, Inc.

9 McKenzie, B.C. (1997) *Medicine and the Internet – Introducing Online Resources and Terminology.* 2nd edition. Oxford: Oxford University Press.

10 Newall, E. (1999) 'Feedback'. [Personal memo to Chellen, S.S]. Available from <ssc1@cant.ac.uk> [Accessed 24 March 1999].

11 Couchman, D. (1999). Research and the Internet. In: *Writer's and Artist's Year Book 1999.* 92nd edition. London: A & C Black.

12 Howe, J. (1998) Referencing the Internet. *Nursing Standard* 13(1) 23–29 Sept.: p. 28.

13 Dwyer, M. (1995) A guide to the Harvard referencing system. In: *British Journal of Nursing* 4(10): pp. 599–602.

14 Bournemouth University Library (1999) Referencing: Harvard system. (www). Available from: <http://www.bournemouth.ac.uk/library/using/harvard_system.html > [Accessed 20 December 2002].

15 Li, X. & Crane, N.B. (1999) *Electronic Styles – A Handbook for Citing Electronic Information.* Medford: Information Today, Inc.

16 British Telecommunications plc (1998) *Home Highway.* London.

17 Central Intelligence Agency Website *The World Factbook 2002.* [online]. Available from: <http://www.odci.gov/cia/publications/factbook/> [Accessed 20 December 2002.]

18 Branscombe, M. (2002) 169 Essential Web design tips. In: *Internet Advisor,* issue 35.

19 Lane, N.D. (1996) *Techniques for Student Research: A Practical Guide.* 2nd edition. Melbourne: Addison Wesley Longman.

Anon (1996) Nurses' Guide to the Internet: purchasing a home computer system and getting connected. In: *AORN Journal*, 64(1): pp. 112–14.

Anthony, D. (1996) Connecting to the Internet. In: *Health Informatics*, 2(2): pp. 78–80.

Arlene Rinaldi (1998) *The Net: User Guidelines and Netiquette.* (WWW). Available from: <http://www.fau.edu/netiquette/net> [Accessed 20 December 2002].

Baskerville, R. (No date) *Netiquette.* [WWW]. Available from <http://www.mcc.ac.uk/~zlsiira/Netiquette/> [Accessed 20 December 2002].

Bowers, L. (1997) Constructing international professional identity: what psychiatric nurses talk about on the Internet. In: *International Journal of Nursing Studies*, 34(3): pp. 208–12.

Fleck, E. (1999) 'Internet support for nurses and midwives'. In: *Professional Nurse*, 14(4): pp. 280–2.

McCue, C. (2000) *Cliffs Notes Exploring the Internet With Yahoo!.* London: IDG Books.

McKibbon, K. (1998) Searching for the best evidence. Part 2: Searching CINAHL, and Medline. In: *Evidence-Based Nursing*, 1(4): pp. 105–7.

Miller, M. (2000) *The Complete Idiot's Guide to Yahoo!.* Indianapolis, IN: Que.

Millhorn, J. (2000) *Student's Companion to the World Wide Web: Social Sciences and Humanities Resources.* Lanham, Maryland: Scarecrow Press.

Monash University (1999) *How to Develop a Search Strategy.* [WWW]. Available from <http://www.lib.monash.edu.au/vl/sstrat/sstrprin.htm> [Accessed 20 December 2002].

Musker, M. (1997) Demystifying the Internet: a guide for nurses. *Nursing Standards*, 12(11): pp. 153–7.

O'Hara, S. (1994) *10 Minute Guide to Buying a Computer.* Indiana: Alpha Books – Macmillan Computer Publishing.

Osbourne, J. (1997) Student Nurses on the Internet. In: *Nursing Standard*, 11(39): p. 49.

Pitcher, M. (1998) Internet sources on leg ulcer management. In: *Journal of Wound Care*, 7(6): pp. 313–16.

Riddlesperger, K. (1996) CINAHL: an exploratory analysis of the current status of nursing theory construction as reflected by the electronic domain. In: *Journal of Advanced Nursing*, 24(3): p. 599.

Ryan, J.M. (1998) A & E Nursing and the Internet. In: *Accident and Emergency Nursing*, 6(2): pp. 106–9.

Tatlow, M.P. (1995) Flexible learning on the information superhighway: FLISH 95. In: *Health Infomatics*, 1(3): pp. 132–6.

Travers, R. (No date) *The Sixteen Commandments of Netiquette.* [Online]. Available from <http://www.argonet.co.uk/zfc/sixt.html> [Accessed 20 December 2002].

Tseng, G., Poulter, A. and Hion, D. (1996) *The Library and Information Professional's guide to the Internet.* London: Library Association Publishing.

Van Lanker, M. (1996) A convert to the net. In: *Nursing Standard*, 10(27): p. 23.

notes

1 Ballard, E. (1996) Getting to grips with it! – Is it worth the effort? In: *CTI Nursing and Midwifery Newsletter* 2(1), Oct. 96: pp.12–13.<http://www.shef.ac.uk/uni/projects/ctinm/newslet/archives/balla.htm> [Accessed January 15th 1998].

2 Howson, N. (1997). What use is the Internet to nurses? In: *CTI Nursing and Midwifery Newsletter* 3(1) Oct. 97: pp. 6–7.

3 Russell, C. (1998) *Internet UK in Easy Steps.* 3rd edition. Warwickshire: Computer Step.

4 Cooper, C. (2001) The Internet and IT for Busy Nurses and Therapists. (WWW). Available from <http://www.carol-cooper.ac.uk/book/> [Accessed: 20 Dec. 2002].

5 Russell, C. (1998) see note 3 above.

6 Lane, N.D. (1996) *Techniques for Student Research: A Practical Guide.* 2nd edition. Addison Wesley Longman. Melbourne.

7 Howson, N. (1997) see note 2 above.

8 Murray, P.J. (1997) Nurses talking online: Who's out there and what are they saying? In: *CTI Nursing and Midwifery Newsletter* 2(3) June 97.

9 Levine, J.R., Young, M.L. and Reinhold, A. (2000) *The Internet for Dummies – Quick Reference.* 6th edition. Forster City: IDG Books Worldwide Inc.

10 Howson, N. (1998) ScHARRP-eyed: What use is the Internet for nurses? keeping current on the net. In: *CTI Nursing and Midwifery Newsletter* 3(3) June 98, pp. 12–13.

11 Russell, C. (1998) see note 3 above.

12 Levine, J.R., Young, M.L. and Reinhold, A. (2000) *The Internet for Dummies – Quick Reference.* 6th edition. IDG Books Worldwide Inc. Forster City.

13 Harmon, C. (1996) *Using the Internet Online Services and CD-ROMs for Writing Research and Term Papers.* New York: Neal-Schuman Publishers, Inc.

14 Tseng, G., Poulter, A. and Hion, D. (1996) *The Library and Information Professional's Guide to the Internet.* London: Library Association Publishing.

15 Russell, C. (1998) see note 3 above.

16 McKenzie, B.C. (1997) *Medicine and the Internet – Introducing Online Resources and Technology.* Oxford: Oxford University Press.

17 Newall, E. (1999) Feedback. [Personal memo to Chellen, S.S.]. Available from <ssc1@cant.ac.uk> [Accessed 24 March 1999].

18 Branscombe, M. (2002) 169 Essential Web design tips. In: *Internet Advisor,* issue 35.

19 Couchman, D. (1999) Research and the Internet. In: *Writer's and Artist's Year Book 1999.* 92nd edition. London: A & C Black.

20 Howe, J. (1998) Referencing the Internet. *Nursing Standard* 13(1) 23–9 Sept, p. 28.

21 Dwyer, M. (1995) A guide to the Harvard referencing system. In: *British Journal of Nursing* 4(10) pp. 599–602.

22 Bournemouth University Library (1999) Referencing: Harvard system. (www). Available from <http://www.bournemouth.ac.uk/library/using/harvard_system.html> [Accessed 20 December 2002].

23 McKenzie, B.C. (1997) see note 16 above.

24 Li, X. and Crane, N.B. (1999) *Electronic Styles – a Handbook for Citing Electronic Information.* Medford: Information Today, Inc.

25 British Telecommunications plc (1998) *Home Highway.* London.

26 Russell, C. (1998) see note 3 above.

27 Central Intelligence Agency Website, *The World Factbook 2002* [online]. Available at <http://www.odci.gov/cia/publications/factbook/> [Accessed 20 December 2002].

index

ENB Healthcare Database, 104, 193
ENTER key, 3
epilepsy, 67, 140
error messages, 136, 183, 219
Eudora, 20, 116, 132
evaluation of resources, 187
evidence-based medicine reviews, 7
evidence-based nursing, 61
Ewan, 167–8
Excite, 36, 82–3, 98, 131
Explore the Virtual Heart, 45

FAQs, 44, 51, 54, 64, 82, 221
favorites, 36, 38–40, 42
fertility, 53
File Transfer protocol, 161, 222
firewalls, 203
first aid sites, 45
flaming, 128, 129, 145
folders, 36, 117, 126, 127, 129
follow-up, 144, 145, 146
formatting text, 177
fpArchie, 165, 166
free access, 11, 52, 64, 161, 210–12
Free Agent, 141
Freeserve, 19, 25, 132, 211, 213
frequently asked questions, *see* FAQs
FrontPage, 181
FTP Explorer, 163
FTP sites, 9, 32, 159–93
    anonymous sites, 160–1, 165
    browser, 162
    dedicated programs, 162–3
    e-mail, 165
    getting web pages on net links, 161
    private sites, 161
    referencing, 193
    session profile, 164
full-duplex card, 158

gateways, 85, 90
getting started, 11, 14, 15, 185
gigabytes, 16
Gopher, 5, 9, 32–3, 69, 159, 166–7, 170, 188, 190, 194
gopherspace, 166
Green Card lottery, 205
Guide to Women's Health Issues, 53

hacker, 13, 203
hard disk, 8, 16, 40, 125, 159, 161, 200–2

hardware, 11, 16, 158, 170, 203
Harmon, 148
Harvard style, 190, 195–6
    internet sources, 192–5
    non-internet sources, 195–6
headers, 39, 117, 119, 131, 138, 141–3, 146–8, 194, 201
heading tags, 174, 177
health care professionals, 69
    journals, 61, 63, 88, 102, 192
    newsgroups, 145
health databases, 41, 104–5
health education, 26, 41
Health Informatics Specialist Group, 67
health information, 5, 10, 43, 52, 65, 71, 199
    Archie, 165–7, 170
    databases, 6, 41, 49, 104–5, 193
    evaluation, 187
    gateways, 46, 72, 88, 86–9, 90–2
    preventative health education web sites, 451–70
    see also journals
Health on the Net, 72, 81
Health Service Journal, 61, 88
health visiting, 26, 41, 52, 69
healthcare research, 26, 41, 59
Healthworks Online, 64
Help desk, 29
help with studies, 6, 7, 9
HENSA, 64
Hepatitis Network, 45
hierarchies, 93, 139, 141
home computer system, 5, 9, 74, 169
    account, 127
    choosing a computer, 15–17
    communication software, 12, 15, 19, 27
    e-mail equipment, 204
    internet service provider, 15, 20–5
    library catalogue searches, 159
    modem, 18
    telephone line, 127, 204
Home Highway, 204
home page, 55
HON, 72, 81, 86, 90–1
hospital trust, 13
hosts, 168
HotBot, 81, *see also* search engines
hotlinks, 31, 33, 38, 40

CL

004.
678
024
61
CHE

5000034917